Healing Arthritis Naturally

WITH ESSENTIAL OIL

Healing Arthritis Naturally

WITH ESSENTIAL OIL

By Rebecca Park Totilo

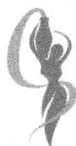

Healing Arthritis Naturally With Essential Oil

Paperback ISBN: 978-0-9991865-3-4
Electronic ISBN: 978-0-9991865-4-1

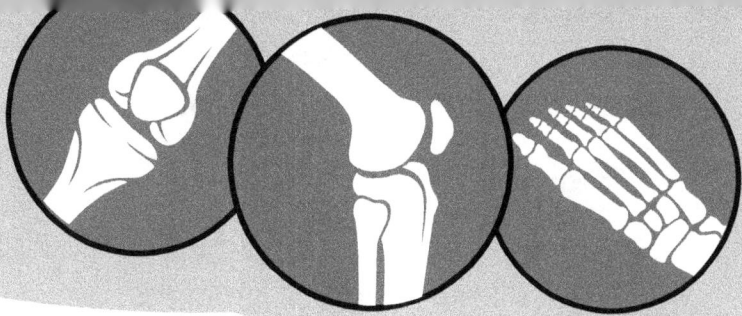

CONTENTS

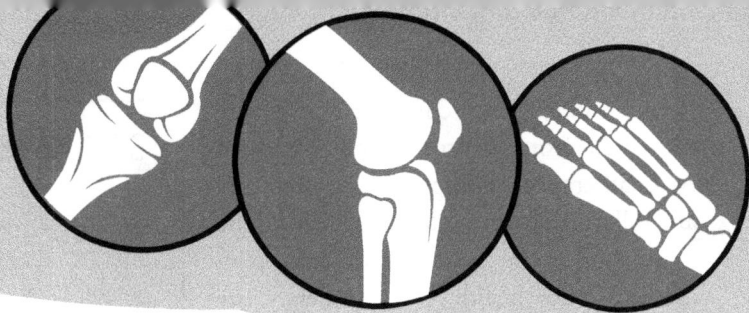

INTRODUCTION

Did you know that arthritis is our nation's leading cause of disability and the most common chronic disease in people over the age of 40? Arthritis affects more than 50 million people nationwide, and this figure is expected to rise to 60 million by 2020, according to the Center for Disease Control.

Arthritis generally afflicts people between the ages of 20 and 50, but all ages can be affected, including infants. The average age for the onset of arthritis is 47 with about three out of every five people having arthritis, under 65 years of age.

The medical community has identified over 100 different forms of arthritis, all sharing one main characteristic: joint inflammation.

If you or someone you love suffers from this crippling disease, nature has provided a remedy: essential oils. Essential oils are a natural and extremely effective way to improve your mobility and quality of life by allieving some of the main symptoms of arthritis, such as pain and swelling.

In this book, we will explore the types and causes of arthritis and which essential oils can offer arthritis relief. More importantly, you will learn how to use essential oils with specific instructions based on the most scientific research.

Please note, the contents here are presented from a professional Certified Aromatherapist standpoint and that any and all health care planning should be made under the guidance of your own medical and health practitioners. The content within only presents an overview of arthritis relief research for educational purposes and does not replace medical advice from a professional physician.

EARLY DETECTION AND TREATMENT IS ESSENTIAL

The two most common types of arthritis are **osteoarthritis (OA)** and **rheumatoid arthritis (RA)**. Although both have similar symptoms, both occur for different reasons. When joints are overused or misused, the results can be OA. In the case of OA, the cushioning cartilage that protects the joint breaks down, resulting in the bones rubbing together. This generally occurs in the knees but can also occur in the hips, spine, and hands (quite often). It is only during the later stages of the disease that a person will most often feel pain, after a significant amount of cartilage is lost.

The second type, rheumatoid arthritis or RA, is a painful inflammatory condition caused by swelling and inflammation of the synovial membrane, the lining of the joint. While this condition is still not fully

DO I HAVE ARTHRITIS?

The signs and symptoms of arthritis vary from person to person. For some, it may be joints cracking suddenly, like knees upon standing. Others may experience stiffness or joints creaking. Maybe pain occurs when twisting a jar open. Early signs can be easily mistaken as an injury or as a result of too much activity. In fact, symptoms may come and go and can be mild to severe. If you have arthritis, you will want to find out early so you can take steps to protect your joints from the permanent damage of uncontrolled inflammation. Early diagnosis and treatment are essential.

By definition, arthritis means "joint inflammation," and the term actually refers to over 100 related conditions or types/forms of the disease. Left untreated it can advance, resulting in joint damage that cannot be undone or reversed.

understood in the medical community, it is classified as an autoimmune disease because it is caused by the body's own immune system attacking the joints. This disorder most often starts in a person's hands, wrists and feet and then advances to shoulders, elbows, and hips. Symptoms for OA and RA include pain, stiffness, fatigue, weakness, slight fever and inflamed tissue lumps under the skin. Also, both OA and RA generally develop symmetrically, i.e., affecting the same joints on both the left and right sides of the body.

Notable differences in OA and RA include **swelling. With RA, people report "soft and squishy" swelling, while people with OA report "hard and bony" swelling.** Another difference is that a person is more likely to develop RA if a parent had it.

Individuals with a history of joint damage, either as a result of an injury or chronic strain, run a higher risk for developing OA.

Arthritic sufferers come in all ages. While it can affect every age group, it seems to focus on those 45 years of age and older. And while neither gender is immune, a reported 74 percent of OA cases (or just over 15 million) occur with women, and a slightly lower percentage of RA cases occur with women.

Weight gain plays a significant role in OA as well. Overweight people tend to develop OA, especially in the knees once they reach 45 years and older. However, the bright side is that losing weight can cut the odds almost in half. Exercise along with regular activity also reduces risk by strengthening joint muscles and reducing joint wear.

Depending on the type and severity of your arthritis, you may experience some of these physical symptoms:

- pain
- stiffness
- tenderness
- swelling
- visible inflammation
- fatigue

> Today, only a small percentage of those afflicted with arthritis become crippled. Most never need canes, wheelchairs, or other ambulatory devices.

Although there isn't a "magic pill" or cure for arthritis, there are a variety of *pain relief treatment strategies including aromatherapy*. Aside from medications, remedies, replacement alternatives, and other helpful treatment options and alternatives, the four main arthritis relief aids are gentle exercises, proper nutrition, an essential oils regimen, and rest. Each of these will be discussed further in subsequent chapters since education plays a significant role in dispelling "old wives' tales" and myths such as "nothing can be done about arthritis."

TRADITIONAL TREATMENTS FOR ARTHRITIS

Allopathic medicine focuses on treatments for arthritis that will improve joint movement and help alleviate pain and inflammation. Your doctor will likely prescribe a combination of treatments that may include different medications and physical therapy before determining which method works best for you. As a last resort, surgery may be necessary for joint repair, joint replacement or fusion.

Medications for arthritis will vary based on the type of arthritis you have. Commonly prescribed medications include:

Analgesics: Over-the-counter pain relievers such as Tylenol, or narcotics such as Percocet, Oxycontin, or Hydrocodone.

Nonsteroidal anti-inflammatory drugs (NSAIDS): Over-the-counter pain relievers and anti-inflammatory meds such as ibuprofen, Advil, Motrin, or Aleve. Others may require a prescription. Some NSAIDs are available in creams or gels that can be rubbed directly on the joints.

Counterirritants: Creams and ointments that contain menthol or capsaicin (the ingredient that makes hot peppers spicy) that can be applied to the skin with hopes of interrupting the pain signals from the affected joint.

Disease-modifying antirheumatic drugs (DMARDs): Medication prescribed for the treatment of rheumatoid arthritis which interrupts the immune system from attacking your affected joints. Examples include methotrexate (Trexall) and hydroxychloroquine (Plaquenil).

Biologic response modifiers: These are used in conjunction with DMARDs to target the proteins that interact with your immune system.

Corticosteroids: Drugs such as prednisone and cortisone are used to reduce inflammation and suppress the immune system. May be taken orally or injected at the site.

TIP: Massage with essential oils is one of the most effective methods of relief found for arthritis. Some believe arthritis can be reversed if diagnosed and treated quickly enough. Managing naturally with essential oils can be extremely helpful in providing relief, making it possible to control the level of pain and the amount of activity you can do.

BASIC SCIENCE OF ARTHRITIS

Joints can handle a lot of heavy pressure. For example, knees feel a force of three to four times a person's total body weight on average just taking a walk. The force of a deep knee bend during a squat can increase to nine times the body weight. So just imagine multiplying the weight of more than 150 pounds times a minimum of three or four, and then even more. That can sure add up to a lot of heavy work on knee joints over time.

Now for the science of this scenario. Where two bones meet, called the **joint**, the bone ends are covered with **cartilage**, also known as **gristle**. This cartilage is sturdy, elastic and spongy or compressible, and keeps the bones from moving against each other at the joint. The cells of this cartilage, called **chondrocytes**, are thought to be the longest living cells of the body.

Surrounding the bones and cartilage is robust and fibrous capsule lined with **synovium,** a thin membrane that lubricates the joint area with fluid. The end result is less friction or smoother rubbing together of the bones. This fluid also feeds the cartilage cells, keeping them healthy, and is "pumped" into them during joint movement. This lack of movement (activity/exercise) can be unhealthy.

Other parts of the body features involved in this arthritic scenario include **muscles, tendons, ligaments, bursae, and mental activity**. Muscles, attached to bones with tendons and ligaments, move bones by contracting. They also cushion movement, absorbing impact or shock. Throughout the muscle and tendon areas are bursae or sacs filled with fluid. These also help cushion movement. And throughout all the coordination of these parts during movement, the brain communicates via nerves throughout the body in particular, the muscles prepare joints for activity.

The exact science of what causes arthritis is still being researched. *For most of the 100-plus forms of arthritis, the causes are unknown.* Injury, overuse of joints and mechanical issues with joints (like skeletal abnormalities, worn out joint muscles) can lead to arthritis. And many point to issues relating to bacteria and germs as some of the problems. Heredity, stress, drugs, food allergies and viruses have also been linked to some forms of arthritis. So have diet, poor circulation and lack of movement.

Essential oils can possibly interact with medications and cause contraindication. Discuss the possible effects with your doctor.

> TIP: Never stop taking any prescribed medications without your healthcare provider's approval. Always discuss your plan of possible reduction and reliance on medications when looking at natural options.

Start slow and watch how your body reacts to the oils. It is recommended to use essential oils approximately four hours following the administration of medications.

LEADING CAUSE OF ARTHRITIS

Arthritic joints can be affected with inflammation when bacteria or a virus (or another undesirable element) enters the joint area or when an injury occurs. What happens is when foreign matter enters this area, or the area sustains an injury, white blood cells, antibodies, and other natural "fighting" mechanisms automatically kick in internally to help. These fighters cause swelling, redness, and heat as the body fluid moves around. Symptoms of inflammation, one of the uncomfortable issues associated with arthritis, are redness, swelling, and tender joints.

MAIN TYPES OF ARTHRITIS

After osteoarthritis (OA) and rheumatoid arthritis (RA), three other major types of arthritis are systemic lupus erythematosus, ankylosing spondylitis, and gout. Let's take a look at each.

Systemic Lupus Erythematosus (SLE) – This form of arthritis mainly affects women. It develops in the skin, internal organs and joints.

Ankylosing Spondylitis – This form of arthritis affects the spine and can also affect the ankles, knees, lungs, heart, shoulders, and eyes.

Gout – This is a painful affliction mainly for men, about one million of them in the United States alone. Uric acid builds up, due to an internal chemical malfunction, forms crystals that get stuck in a joint, generally the big toe, and become inflamed.

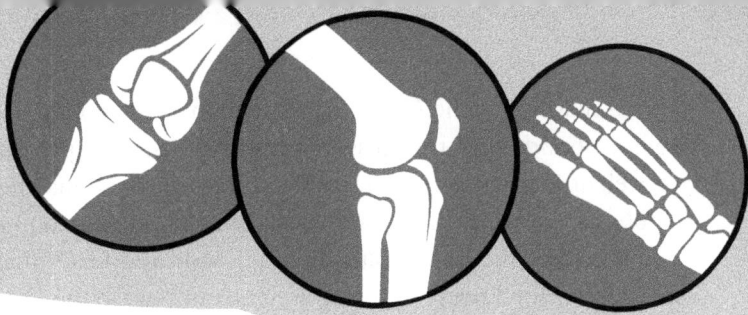

ARTHRITIC OPTIONS TODAY

There are many ways to manage arthritic pain today to find relief. Available are arthritic diets, exercise programs, over-the-counter and prescription medications, relaxation and positive emotion coping techniques. Other options available include surgeries, supplements, home remedies, and natural alternative therapies.

When arthritis is first suspected, it would be wise to seek a medical opinion first. Then as time and resources allow, check out the other options. The basics of each follow.

ARTHRITIC DIETS AND NUTRITIONAL HEALING

While diet doesn't cure arthritis, certain foods have been shown to reduce inflammation, strengthen bones and boost the immune system. So, overall dietary changes for health is essential and comes into play. Obesity and weight gain can also affect certain arthritic conditions, putting additional stress on weight-bearing joints. According to the Arthritis Foundation, every pound of excess weight exerts about 4 pounds of extra pressure on the knees. So a person who is 10 pounds overweight is placing 40 pounds of extra pressure on his knees; a person who is 50 pounds overweight has 200 pounds of extra pressure on his knees. This added weight stresses the joints, causing more wear and tear, inflammation and pain, especially in the knees. So losing weight can reduce the inflammatory response and significantly lower inflammation in the body. Eatting a healthy diet and seeking guidance from your healthcare provider to assist you in setting up and following a well-balanced dietary plan is advised.

To begin, here is a look at some vitamins, minerals, nutrients/foods, and herbal applications to consider.

VITAMINS

Vitamin B5 – When grouped and tanked together, B vitamins work at their peak. They, and B5 specifically, are useful for reducing swelling.

Vitamin B3 – This vitamin reduces tissue swelling and dilates small arteries, increasing blood flow. Note that Vitamin B3 is NOT advised for persons with high blood pressure, gout or liver disorders.

Vitamin B6 – Another B that reduces tissue swelling.

Vitamin B12 – This vitamin aids in multiple functions. It helps with cell formation, digestion, myelin production, and nerve protection.

Vitamin C – This vitamin acts as an anti-inflammatory, relieves pain, and rids the body of free radicals.

Vitamin E – This is a potent antioxidant that protects joints from free radicals while increasing joint flexibility.

Vitamin K – This vitamin assists with a mineral deposit into the bone matrix.

MINERALS

Boron – This trace mineral aids in bone health.

Calcium – This is a much-needed mineral for bone health.

Magnesium – Magnesium helps keep calcium in balance within the body.

Zinc – This mineral is necessary for bone growth, but is often lacking in arthritic patients.

Manganese – Manganese is also necessary for bone growth. However, do not ingest manganese with calcium because they can work against each other.

Copper – Copper helps to strengthen connective tissue.

Germanium – This antioxidant helps with pain relief.

Sulfur – A lack of sulfur can result in deterioration of ligaments, cartilage, collagen, and tendons.

NUTRIENT COMBOS

Chondroitin Sulfate – This lubrication in joints, joint fluid, and connective tissue can be found in the sea cucumber.

Gelatin – This cheap source helps with raw cartilage replenishing.

Glucosamine Sulfate – This combo is necessary for tendon, ligament, bone, cartilage, and synovial (joint) fluid formation.

Quercetin – This helps with inflammation reduction.

Type II Collagen – Use this for the growth and repair of joints, articular cartilage, and connective tissue.

OTHER FACTORS

There are many factors to consider with regards to arthritic diets and nutritional healing, and each factor may not apply to each individual. For example, certain people are allergic to specific foods, and these allergies can indeed worsen arthritic conditions.

Ingesting foods that contain sodium nitrate or tartrazine can inflame rheumatoid arthritis while ingesting foods containing a substance called hydrazine can contribute to systemic lupus erythematosus, an arthritic condition connected to lupus. There is a rare type of arthritis called Behcet's Disease, and eating black walnuts can cause flare-ups in people with this rare condition. So as you see, there is a variety of arthritic conditions and along with them a variety of foods that may trigger them. The best way to approach the situation is to examine each arthritic condition and tailor one's approach based upon the specifics.

There is a prevalence of people living with rheumatoid arthritis that have an abnormally low blood zinc level. Several independent studies have been conducted where rheumatoid arthritis patients have been given increased doses of zinc and showed marginal improvement, yet the tests were not extensive enough to be conclusive. The effects of copper on rheumatoid arthritis have been studied for a long time,

> When treating joint pain caused by arthritis the first thing to do is look at your diet. Decrease your intake of simple carbohydrates and avoid coffee and red meat. Increase your vegetables, fruits, complex carbohydrates, wheat germ, and oily fish.

and although results vary there seems to be some case for using copper to improve the condition, although most of the medical profession has dismissed this therapy as relatively ineffective. Copper therapy is not discouraged, however, when approached from food sources and may work on some individuals. It is suggested that if you do attempt copper therapy, that copper-rich foods are utilized instead of copper supplements, since copper supplements can cause side effects which include change in the sense of taste and smell, nausea, vomiting, loss of appetite, abnormal blood clots, increased joint pain, chills, anemia, and kidney problems. Also, excess copper can cause cirrhosis of the liver in patients prone to Wilson's Disease. Check with your doctor to be sure you are not inclined to storing excess copper in your body. There is an extensive choice of foods you can enjoy in order to increase your copper intake: lamb; pork; pheasant quail; duck; goose; squid; salmon; organ meats including liver, heart, kidney, brain; shellfish including oysters, scallops, shrimp, lobster, clams, and crab; meat gelatin; soy protein meat substitutes; tofu; nuts and seeds; chocolate milk; soy milk; cocoa. These are just a few of the foods that are rich in copper.

As for foods to avoid when suffering from rheumatoid arthritis, many nutritionists and naturopaths suggest avoiding dairy products altogether, as they seem to exacerbate rheumatoid arthritis flare-ups. Because of the risk in overdosing, one should be discouraged from taking doses of vitamins that are higher than recommended without a physician's direction. Some vitamins and minerals can worsen certain conditions, and the concentration that can be attained through vitamins can be dangerous. It is much better to approach any desired increase in vitamin or mineral intake through food therapy.

There has been some success with the food supplements glucosamine and chondroitin in relieving symptoms of pain and stiffness for some persons with osteoarthritis. These supplements can be found in pharmacies and health food stores; however, the purity of the products or the dose of the active ingredients cannot be specified because the FDA does not monitor these supplements. The National Institutes of Health is studying glucosamine and chondroitin, so more should be known about the effectiveness of these products for osteoarthritis in the near future. Patients with osteoarthritis taking blood-thinners should be careful taking chondroitin as it can increase blood-thinning and cause excessive bleeding. Fish oil supplements have been shown to have some anti-inflammation properties and increasing the dietary fish intake and/or fish oil capsules (Omega-3 capsules) can sometimes reduce inflammation of arthritis. With osteoarthritis there is also the concern with the deterioration of cartilage; therefore those with osteoarthritis should avoid large doses of vitamin-A since there is some evidence that it contributes to cartilage deterioration. In the case of fibromyalgia, although clinical proof is once again sparse, there are a lot of personal experiences of improvement of this condition when certain dietary practices are followed. Eliminating wheat, dairy, citrus, sugar, aspartame, alcohol, caffeine, and tobacco seem to be universal in those that have had success in treating the illness through dietary means. According to Dr. Joseph Mercola, author of "The Total Health Program," nine of ten sufferers of fibromyalgia are female, and 76% of those who followed suggested dietary rules experienced a significant reduction in pain. The thing to keep in mind with fibromyalgia is that, unlike the other common arthritis ailments, it is more of a syndrome than a disease, and much of it can be reversed. Making corrections to diet as well as reducing stress and getting plenty of rest can lead to a full recovery.

HERBAL AND OTHER NATURAL AND HOME REMEDIES AND SUPPLEMENTS

For people who have arthritis, dependable pain relief is a vital concern. The agonizing sensations of simply walking up the stairs are discouraging and can drive patients into depression. When someone cannot function properly, their body is not in balance; often, they will become victims of their pain, forcing them to seek alternatives. These people have often tried traditional medications without success, they are often not eligible for surgery, and as a result, they will seek relief through natural remedies.

Many people are also seeking natural remedies because of the increasing cost of prescription medication. Before discontinuing a prescription drug, consult a physician. However, with a doctor's approval, there are many natural solutions, which may aid in managing arthritis.

TIP: Cayenne Cream

Apply the cayenne cream to painful areas. Cayenne peppers contain a substance called capsaicin which is responsible for their spicy effect. This also causes a burning sensation when it comes in contact with skin, and inhibits the body's production of substance P, which is heavily involved in relaying signals of pain to the brain. Apply the cream two to three times a day for at least one week before deciding whether or not the cream is helping to reduce arthritis pain.

It's understandable that many people reach for the aspirin or another pain reliever when experiencing pain and achy joints due to osteoarthritis. The problem is that these medications can be rough on your stomach, and they do nothing to slow the progression of your arthritis. Even the new COX-2 inhibitor drugs do not act to preserve the joint (from the doctors of WholeHealthMD).

On the contrary, many natural remedies and supplements have been found to actually reduce cartilage deterioration and even rebuild a patient's lost cartilage. However, before adding any to your daily routine, check with your healthcare advisor, as supplements can cause adverse reactions and may not be right for your situation. Note that dietary supplements are not regulated by the FDA (Food and Drug Administration); i.e., they do not need to be approved by them, and can include any of the following: plants, fats, proteins, animal organs and tissues as well as herbs, minerals, and vitamins. So some supplements may be fine for arthritic patients; however, some may not be. Note also that manufacturers may very well promote that their products work great, but they do not have to use standardized ingredients or recipes, disclose side effects that have been reported, nor prove that the products are indeed effective. Since supplements are not FDA-approved they must be accompanied by a two-part disclaimer on the product label: that the statement has not been evaluated by FDA and that the product is not intended to "diagnose, treat, cure or prevent any disease." So use caution.

The most popular dietary supplements for arthritis sufferers are **chondroitin, fish oil and glucosamine**. Chondroitin draws fluid into the cartilage, improving shock-absorbing ability and weight control (as more weight equals more joint pressure).

Fish oil helps with controlling inflammation in the body. And recent studies have shown that the cartilage-building substance called **glucosamine** is effective for the long-term relief of osteoarthritis pain. In some people, glucosamine appears even to slow the deterioration of joints over time and reinforce joint cartilage. Whether or not it can reverse the disease is still unclear. In some instances, glucosamine can be used in conjunction with MSM, a substance that appears to slow down the degeneration but is not yet proven and approved.

In a nutshell:

- **Chondroitin** – Helps draw fluid into cartilage, improving shock-absorbing ability.

- **Ginger** – Ginger is an antioxidant that acts as an inflammatory with no significant side effects.

- **Glucosamine sulfate** – This builds cartilage with very few side effects.

- **Magnets** – Although magnets that are worn as jewelry or placed on bed linens have been reported by some to be effective pain relievers, results are still preliminary; doctors claim that these magnets are not strong enough.

- **MSM** – This organic sulfur is used in the reduction of inflammation.

- **Nettle Leaf** – Nettle leaf can reduce a patient's need for NSAIDs (non-steroidal anti-inflammatory drugs) by up to 70 percent.

- **Vitamin E** – This antioxidant is used primarily for osteoarthritis.

- **Vitamin B** – This is an effective pain reliever. It works best on the knee and can help stop degeneration that is caused by free-radical molecules, not only in the joints but other areas of the body as well.

While these are just a few examples of what a person living with arthritis can use when seeking pain relief from natural supplements, due to the lack of scientific study and testing on many of these alternative treatments, there is little proof of their effectiveness.

Doctors claim nothing can cure osteoarthritis, but nutritional supplements, the application of heat or cold to affected joints, exercise, and weight loss can improve the function and flexibility of your joints, and perhaps even slow the progress of the disease.

Conventional over-the-counter pain relievers, such as acetaminophen and ibuprofen, can be very helpful in decreasing joint pain, but they do produce side effects and can cause problems in long-term users. Could essential oils be the answer? In the next few chapters, we will be exploring the benefits of essentials oils for people living with arthritis.

TIP: Ginger Tea

Ginger is one of nature's most potent anti-inflammatory medicinal roots that has been used for thousands of years. Steep two tablespoons of grated fresh ginger in a quart of water and sip this throughout the day for joint pain relief.

EXERCISE AND MOVEMENT FOR ARTHRITIS SUFFERERS

Exercise can be very beneficial for people living with arthritis, often relieving stiffness in joints and strengthening muscles, thereby reducing stress on joints, keeping bone and cartilage tissue strong and healthy, and increasing flexibility. A recommended 30-minute minimum of daily activity is the norm. Before starting any exercise program, it is vital that you speak to their doctor to ensure there are no hidden risks. However, you will find that most doctors recommend exercise for their arthritis patients either on their own initiative or when asked.

The types of exercises suggested vary; however, with all types of exercise, the warm-up is the starting point. Warming up is best started with applying warm compresses to the joints, followed by mild stretching. The range-of-motion exercises, such as dance, is a perfect start, as are low-impact aerobics. These can relieve stiffness and increase flexibility. Never discount the effectiveness of walking as an exercise. Walking is a great exercise to improve the arthritic condition, and carrying weights as light as one pound and using your arms as you walk can involve the whole body. The "trick" is to make walking interesting enough as an exercise to stay motivated. Try walking in different settings, alternating walking with dance on different days, and of course including a partner can be much more interesting than going at it alone.

Aquatics: Exercising in a pool is a great way to exercise as well. Water is an excellent aid because it provides resistance that builds muscle in the entire body while reducing shock to the joints at the same time. Additionally, because the whole body tends to become involved in aquatic exercise the added benefit of cardiovascular exercise is enjoyed. If at all possible, find a heated pool to work out in. Warm water is soothing to the joints and will cause the blood vessels to dilate, increasing circulation. With that in mind, it is often beneficial to add using a spa to your regimen, perhaps after your workout, to provide some soothing jets of

There are two types of pain—acute and chronic—which affect the systems of the body. Acute in general refers to pain that will end; pain caused by burns, broken bones, headaches, etc. Chronic, on the other hand, refers to pain that is persistent, wearing and gets worse with time rather than better—arthritis, for example. Arthritis attacks the joints, quite often the hands due to their complex arrangement of joints, bones, and tendons.

water to your muscles and even more help with increased circulation, which is always vital when dealing with arthritis.

Yoga: If you still want more variety, you may want to try yoga. Yoga is a general term for several stretching and pose-oriented exercises originating in India and is incredibly beneficial toward achieving flexibility and reducing stress physically and mentally. There are gentle forms of yoga such as Hatha Yoga that are excellent to start with. Hatha Yoga comprises of gentle stretches and simple poses that help flexibility and balance, and are easy to learn and enjoy. Check your local activities paper or section of your local newspaper to see if there are any yoga classes near you.

Even when you cannot make it out to walk or to an aquatics or yoga class, **there are exercises you can do daily to improve flexibility, strength, and conditioning**. You can flex your legs while sitting in a chair facing forward, just by moving your leg outward while keeping your foot on the floor and holding it there for a few seconds, then retracting it until your foot is behind you, then alternating to the other leg. Interlocking your fingers and slowly flexing your wrists to the left and the right for a few minutes a day can help tremendously to increase flexibility and reduce pain in the wrist area.

For your upper back, you can stand upright in front of a table, then lean over and place your hands on the table and tuck your chin back toward your collarbone. Once positioned as such, lift your upper back upward and simultaneously take a deep breath. Hold that position for 5-10 seconds and then relax while exhaling. While doing this, lower your spine slowly as you move both shoulder blades forward as if toward each other. Repeat this exercise for 10-15 repetitions.

For the shoulders and middle back, start again from an upright position standing as straight as you can, reach back and lock the fingers of both hands together. Breathe slowly and deeply and lift upward with your shoulders while exhaling at the same time. Be sure to keep your chest up and your chin in. Repeat this for about 10-15 sets.

For the shoulders and upper chest, choose a free corner of the room to stand in and place your hands on the opposite sides of the corner. Take a step back about 18 inches from the edge. You now should be facing the corner directly with your hands on both of the walls with your body some distance from the wall itself. Keeping your chest up after inhaling, lean in toward the corner while exhaling. Repeat this exercise for 10-15 sets.

Whatever exercise program you choose, **be sure to breathe properly when exercising**. Oxygenation is vital to any exercise regimen as it promotes a healthy heart rate and reduces fatigue; additionally, oxygenation helps circulation, which is critical for achieving the flexibility and strength that you are trying to accomplish in battling arthritis. Also, listen to your body. It is natural to feel a little fatigue and soreness when starting a new exercise regimen, However, if the pain of soreness persists for more than one hour, or you have a decrease in mobility that lasts longer than an hour, then the regimen should be reduced until the soreness desists. Also, look for signs of increased swelling of joints or any persistent increase of weakness; these are signs of activities that are too strenuous and a reduction in activity will be necessary. Just remember to take all new exercise regimens slowly at the start. The idea is to increase flexibility, not train for the Olympics.

There are three main types of exercises to include in a basic exercise program:

Range-of-motion exercises – These lessen stiffness and help with improving flexibility. "Range of motion" refers to the area within which the joints move naturally or on a daily basis. Although these range-of-motion exercises can be performed every day, it is recommended that they are only done every other day.

Strengthening exercises – There are two types of strengthening exercises; isometric or tightening the muscles without moving the joints, and isotonic, moving of the joints for strengthening muscle movements. It is recommended to do these sets of exercises every other day unless you are suffering from more than mild joint pain or swelling.

Endurance exercises – The objective of these is to increase stamina. They also help with improving your inner personal/mental strength as well as weight control and sleep. Some of the most popular endurance exercises are bike riding, walking, and water exercising. These are great if you only suffer from mild joint pain or swelling. A twenty to thirty-minute workout or two to three short 10-minute bouts during the day is recommended about three times each week.

Let's sum up exercise with a few tips:

- Establish your own unique, exercise program that meets your personal health needs, budget, and environment. Make sure it is safe by checking with your healthcare provider or workout trainer. Take it slow and steady like Aesop's turtle in the race.

- Be kind to yourself. Stop if something hurts. You may want to apply heat before exercising and doing warm up to prevent injury. Be sure to cool off afterward with ice packs.

- Enjoy exercising by making it a routine during the week. Include range-of-motion, strengthening and endurance exercises as part of your regimens. Also, vary your activities by trying a new class at a health club once every quarter. Try joining a naturalist group for weekly hikes in local parks. Check local newspapers, library bulletin boards, postings at gyms and clubs, etc. for healthy activities like walk-a-thons and bike-a-thons for nonprofits. You'll meet new friends, have fun, get out more and exercise all at the same time.

- Instructional pilates or yoga classes are available free on the internet. No need for spending time and money elsewhere. You can watch videos online or borrow exercise DVDs from the local public library. Get active by washing windows, cleaning your house, car, pet, children's closets, your closets, anything – just get moving.

TIP: Swimming regularly is an excellent exercise for people living with arthritis. This helps keep your joints supple.

RELAXATION AND COPING TIPS

The importance of relaxation in controlling and treating disease, in general, has only recently been recognized throughout the medical industry, yet its implementation still lags, and the general public still does not understand its effectiveness. Relaxation techniques, especially those involving meditation, have been seen as a bunch of "mumbo-jumbo" for many years until the findings of scientists and doctors that showed immense benefits to this practice became more prevalent. Relaxation techniques have a definite place in the healing process of the body, and with arthritis, the case is no different. With certain types of arthritis, the importance of relaxation is increased, since stress and emotional disposition play a large part in them.

Prayer is a form of relaxation and meditation if you are spiritually or religiously inclined that works wonders. Either following a minister or someone else leading prayer, or formulating your own inspirational prayer, you can call upon God and seek his comfort, as you see him taking your pain away. Again, mental and physical benefits are realized from such a practice.

You may also consider hypnosis as an option. Hypnosis is just a guided meditation that allows you to access the power of your subconscious mind through a guide called a hypnotist, who is either a trained psychologist, psychiatrist, counselor, or social worker. Images of a man with a shiny gold stopwatch putting you under a trance to make you perform unusual acts or reveal deep dark secrets are more the scripts of Hollywood movies than what real-life hypnotism is. In the case of hypnosis for pain management, hypnosis is nothing more than an assisted guided imagery, such as described above. The only difference here is that you have someone to help you through the steps of relaxation and meditation on your image.

Yoga is another modality that is very beneficial both for flexibility as well as relaxation. Forms of yoga such as Bhakta are devotional while Raja is meditation-oriented. They can provide a great deal of healing toward all types of arthritis.

OTHER WAYS TO HELP REDUCE INFLAMMATION

There are other ways to help decrease inflammation in the body that can be used in conjunction with essential oils. Using these different methods together with essential oils will help to speed up healing time while reducing inflammation and infection.

- Try increasing your vitamins and minerals such as zinc, vitamin D, and Omega-3s.
- Try introducing probiotics into your diet.
- Try eating healthier with more organic foods.
- Reduce your intake of trans-fats.
- Get a massage.
- Eat more anti-inflammatory spices such as ginger, turmeric, and oregano.
- Cut down on your refined sugar intake.
- Get more antioxidants into your diet.
- Exercise more regularly.
- Try yoga and meditation.
- Drink more fluids to help the body get rid of harmful toxins.
- Apply ice to the affected areas to help reduce pain and swelling.
- Diffuse oils like lavender, bergamot, lemon, and Roman chamomile to help uplift the spirit, these work as antidepressants.

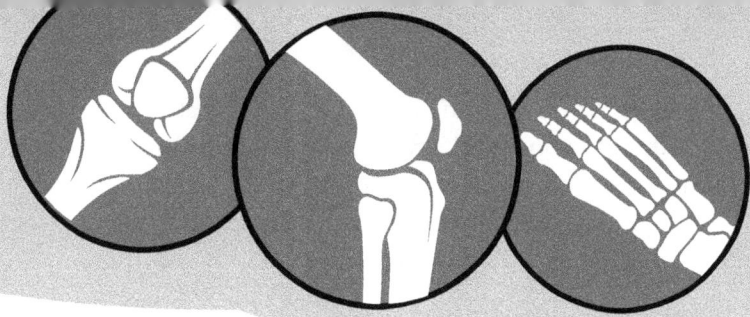

WHAT IS AN ESSENTIAL OIL?

Before examining how essential oils can help with arthritis, let's first look at what an essential oil is and how it works. Essential oils are a fragrant, vital fluid distilled from flowers, shrubs, leaves, trees, roots, and seeds. Because they are necessary for the life of the plant and play a vital role in the biological processes of the vegetation, these substances are called "essential." They carry the lifeblood, intelligence, and vibrational energy that endow them with the healing power to sustain their own life—and help the people who use them.

TIP: Before using essential oils for any health condition, be sure to study each essential oils' profile to learn how each one works in general, as well as learn about their unique characteristics.

Since essential oils are derived from a natural plant source, you will notice that the oil does not leave an "oily" or greasy spot. Unlike fatty vegetable oils used for cooking (composed of molecules too large to penetrate at a cellular level), essential oils are a non-greasy liquid consisting of tiny molecules that can permeate every cell and administer healing at the most fundamental level of our body. Their unique chemical makeup allows them to pass through the skin and the cell membranes where most needed. Whether diffused into the air or applied to the skin, they immediately are absorbed and go straight to action and can perform various functions.

Essential oils come from aromatic plants and their parts including trees, grasses, fruit, leaves, flowers, bark, needles, roots, and seeds. All essential oils have unique medicinal properties, characteristics and therapeutic benefits that will differ depending on the soil, climate, and altitude of the countries where the plants were grown.

Plant substances that have been extracted into essential oils are used in aromatherapy to promote well-being and good health. While the term aromatherapy can seem ambiguous, "scent" is only one aspect of aromatherapy, as you will discover many more dramatic benefits for healing the body, mind, and spirit.

Many people have reported authentic healing when using them—though everyone may not experience the same results as family history, lifestyle, and diet plays a significant role in the body's healing process. Essential oils work together in harmony, making them inherently safe, unlike when multiple prescription drugs are taken, causing drug-interaction.

ESSENTIAL OILS FOR ARTHRITIS

If you're are looking for a natural alternative to treating your arthritis symptoms as opposed to over-the-counter (OTC) or prescription medications, essential oils may be your answer.

Aromatherapy is one of the fastest growing fields in alternative medicine for arthritis used in the home, as well as in clinical and hospital environments. Certain essential oils have been shown to reduce significant symptoms, such as pain, stiffness, inflammation, and anxiety.

Becoming familiar with the qualities and common benefits of essential oils for arthritis will give you the confidence in using oils for wellness within the body.

Whether it's achy joints, sore muscles or something more serious, essential oils can help ease pain and reduce swelling caused by arthritis. Modern medicine now believes that the nation's leading diseases such as heart disease, diabetes, and arthritis are all linked to one problem: inflammation. Essential oils offer us a natural remedy for reducing and preventing inflammation for these various conditions in the body.

As you will see in the following charts, there are many benefits to using essential oils to help your body eliminate inflammatory wastes, improve circulation and speed up the recovery time. The essential oils listed contain several of the chemical constituents researched by the scientific and medical community for the relief of symptoms of OA and RA, with each having its own set of benefits depending on the chemical constituents each is composed of.

Some of the therapeutic properties found in these essential oils are documented as being antispasmodic, anti-inflammatory, analgesic (pain-relieving) and much more. When applied topically, the oil will easily penetrate the skin and can be carried through the bloodstream to affected areas where you need it most within minutes.

Aromatherapy is a very effective holistic treatment used by some arthritic sufferers for pain relief and stress management. Treatment focuses on using pleasurable aromatic botanical oils by either massaging them into the skin, adding them to the bath water, inhaling them directly or diffusing their scents into the surrounding environment. The oils you choose to use for blends will not only help with relaxation but will lessen pain via olfactory nerve stimulation when inhaled.

Essential oils' chemical constituents that have therapeutic potential as dietary supplements include linalool and linalyl acetate. These particular compounds are known to reduce and eliminate inflammation and lessen pain in the body. An example of a few oils that contain these constituents include bergamot, lavender, eucalyptus, and marjoram, all having linalyl acetate in high amounts. There are many other, though; in fact, over 200 plants produce linalool.

Sometimes with arthritic pain, heat can help. Essential oils that have rubefacient effects such as black pepper, clove bud, or ginger can help with their warming effect. These can be added to other essential oils that have analgesic and anti-inflammatory actions.

Oils such as birch and wintergreen are the only plants in the world that naturally contain methyl salicylate and have been documented as having cortisone-like effects that can relieve pain quickly. These, and peppermint as well, offer a cooling effect.

Another favorite oil, frankincense can inhibit the production of inflammation associated with conditions like arthritis and help prevent the breakdown of the cartilage tissue.

Essential oils such as oregano, marjoram, thyme, and rosemary are high in carvacrol, a phenol that can be very effective as a natural anti-inflammatory. This compound acts in the same way as common anti-arthritis drugs by inhibiting an inflammatory enzyme known as COX-2.

Essential oils that increase blood circulation and have a warming effect, acting as natural muscle relaxers, include basil, cypress, marjoram, rosemary, chamomile, clary sage, lavender, and wintergreen to name a few. With so many oils possessing these properties, you will see some overlap in their benefits and uses.

Ginger, which has been used traditionally as an anti-inflammatory remedy for centuries, contains an active chemical constituent called gingerol. A study in 2006 revealed that its phenolic secondary metabolites were consistent with these traditional uses as a potent anti-arthritic compound for rheumatoid arthritis and streptococcal cell wall (SCW)-induced arthritis. The Arthritis Foundation reported on another study conducted at the University of Miami their findings that "ginger extract could be a substitute to nonsteroidal anti-inflammatory drugs (NSAIDS)."

TIP: For rheumatoid arthritis try combining a couple of drops of birch and oregano oils in a carrier oil such as coconut oil to reduce rheumatic pain. For sharp RA pain, use lavender and marjoram essential oils.

Basil is used in relieving muscular aches and pains, colds and flu, hay fever, asthma, bronchitis, mental fatigue, anxiety, and depression. It is incredibly soothing and uplifting and is popular with massage therapists for alleviating tension and stress in their patients. When applied in dilution, basil is reputed as having anti-inflammatory effects due to its chemical constituents 1,8-cineole that reduces swelling and linalool, a compound that diminishes edema, lessening the risk of cartilage damage. It is also highly useful as an antispasmodic, as well as an antiemetic, antiseptic, carminative, cephalic, expectorant, and immune support. It is loaded with antioxidant, anti-inflammatory actions. This oil may irritate sensitive skin. Avoid use during pregnancy. Usage: oral, topical, inhalation. **Note:** Top

Benzoin has a sweet, warm, vanilla-like aroma. Its main constituent is benzoic acid, which has properties that are antiseptic, antidepressant, anti-inflammatory, carminative, deodorant, diuretic, and expectorant. The sweet resin is widely used medicinally for respiratory ailments and skin conditions such as acne, eczema, and psoriasis. Benzoin is non-toxic and non-irritant but is a mild sensitizer and should be avoided if you have allergy-prone skin. Usage: topical, inhalation. **Note:** Base

Bergamot is used in many skin care creams and lotions because of its refreshing and citrusy nature. It is ideal for helping to calm inflamed skin and is an ingredient in some creams for eczema and psoriasis. Bergamot's chemical makeup has antiseptic properties, which help ward off infection and aid recovery. It is a favorite oil of aromatherapists in treating depression. Bergamot is also useful as an antispasmodic and helps to reduce leg cramps and is used for restless leg syndrome. It is also suitable for coughs and works as a digestive aid. The therapeutic properties of bergamot include analgesic, antidepressant, antiseptic, antibiotic, antispasmodic, stomachic, calmative, cicatrizant, deodorant, digestive, febrifuge, vermifuge, and vulnerary. As a natural antibiotic with antiseptic properties, it can help reduce and eliminate infections associated with inflammation. It also relieves the pain that is associated with inflammation. Bergamot's sedative property helps the body to relax and heal, with its antispasmodic property helps to calm the muscles while increasing blood flow and circulation to promote a quicker healing time. Bergamot essential oil has phototoxic properties. Therefore, exposure to the sun must be avoided after use. It may also interfere with the activity of certain prescription drugs (NSAIDs, proton-pump inhibitors, acetaminophen, antiepileptics, immune modulators, blood-sugar medications, blood pressure medications, antidepressants, antipsychotics, diabetic medications, antihistamines, antibiotics, and anesthetics). Usage: oral, topical, inhalation. **Note:** Top

Birch has a sweet, sharp, camphoraceous scent that is fresh and similar to wintergreen. It is credited with analgesic, anti-inflammatory, antirheumatic, antiseptic, astringent, depurative, diuretic and tonic properties. Birch is a valuable addition to many massage oil blends for sore muscles, sprains, and painful joints because of these anti-inflammatory and antispasmodic properties. Birch essential oil is potentially toxic and may cause skin irritation. Avoid use with epileptics or children under 12. Dilute properly and avoid during pregnancy or lactation. Do not use orally. May interact with aspirin, blood pressure, antiplatelet, and anticoagulant medications, and increase the risk of bleeding among those who suffer from bleeding disorders. Avoid if allergic to aspirin, methyl salicylate, or other NSAIDs. Usage: topical, inhalation. **Note:** Top

Black Pepper is used in the treatment of pain, rheumatism, chills, flu, colds, nausea, poor circulation, exhaustion, muscular aches and for stimulating the appetite. Black pepper is a potent anti-inflammatory agent. Its properties include analgesic, antiseptic, antispasmodic, anti-toxic, aphrodisiac, antiemetic, antiviral, digestive, diuretic, anti-inflammatory, expectorant, febrifuge, rubefacient, and warming. This oil may irritate sensitive skin and if used too much could over-stimulate the kidneys. May interfere with the enzymes responsible for drug metabolism (NSAIDs, proton-pump inhibitors, acetaminophen, antiepileptics, antidepressants, antipsychotics, diabetic medications, antihistamines, antibiotics, and anesthetics.) Usage: oral, topical, inhalation. **Note:** Middle-Base

Camphor, White is known to be clarifying, energizing, and purifying. The chemical constituents of camphor are anti-inflammatory, antiseptic, carminative, diuretic, insecticide, and laxative properties. Camphor has been used in the treatment of inflammation, arthritis, muscular aches and pains, sprains, rheumatism, bronchitis, coughs, colds, fever, flu, and infectious diseases. Its anti-inflammatory and analgesic properties work together to reduce pain and inflammation present in the body. Camphor's sedative properties are essential in helping to relieve inflammation, as it allows the body to relax and rest, promoting healing. Camphor oil is a powerful oil and should be used with caution. Overdosing can cause convulsions and vomiting. Pregnant women or persons who have epilepsy and asthma should not use it. Avoid with children under six due to high camphor content. Do not take orally. Usage: topical. **Note:** Top

Cedarwood assists with acne, arthritis, dandruff, and dermatitis. Cedarwood is helpful for the respiratory system, elimination of excess phlegm and catarrh. It fights urinary tract infections, as well as bladder and kidney disorders while improving oily skin. The therapeutic properties of Cedarwood are anti-seborrheic, antiseptic, antispasmodic, anti-inflammatory, tonic, circulatory stimulant, antirheumatic, astringent, diuretic, emmenagogue, expectorant, insecticide, sedative and fungicidal. Cedarwood supports a normal inflammatory response by inhibiting the 5-LOX enzyme (in vitro). It is considered a non-toxic and non-irritant oil. Himalayan cedarwood reduces inflammation and autoimmune disorders such as rheumatoid arthritis. Usage: oral, topical, inhalation. **Note:** Base

Chamomile, German is a relaxing and rejuvenating agent that calms nerves, reduces stress and aids with insomnia. Chamomile is known for its anti-inflammatory abilities and can help in alleviating muscle spasms and joint pain. It can assist with cuts, wounds and insect bites and works as an excellent skin cleanser. Chamomile is nourishing for dry and itchy skin, eases puffiness and strengthens tissues. German chamomile is known to smooth out broken capillaries, thus improving skin elasticity. Chamomile is also high in anti oxidants which can help rid the body of harmful toxins that may be present in the area of inflammation. Its therapeutic properties include analgesic, anti-allergic, anti-convulsive, antidepressant, antiseptic, antispasmodic, anti-inflammatory, cholagogue, diuretic, emmenagogue, febrifuge, hepatic, nervine, sedative, splenetic, stomachic, sudorific, tonic, vermifuge, and vasoconstrictor. Azulene gives this oil its intense blue color, while sesquiterpenes lend its calming effect. While German chamomile is considered non-toxic and non-irritant, it could cause dermatitis in some individuals. Do not use this essential oil during pregnancy because it is a uterine stimulant. Avoid this oil if you suffer from allergies to ragweed. Usage: oral, topical, inhalation. **Note:** Middle

Chamomile, Roman is effective for skin care for most skin types, acne, allergies, boils, burns, eczema, inflamed skin conditions, wounds, menstrual pain, premenstrual syndrome, headache, insomnia, restless leg syndrome, and nervous tension. The therapeutic properties of Roman chamomile oil are analgesic, antispasmodic, antiseptic, antibiotic, anti-inflammatory, anti-infectious, antidepressant, antineuralgic, antiphlogistic, antiseptic, bactericidal, carminative, cholagogue, cicatrizant, emmenagogue, febrifuge, hepatic, sedative, nervine, digestive, tonic, sudorific, stomachic, vermifuge and vulnerary. It is non-toxic and non-irritant. This oil should not be used by anyone who is allergic to ragweed. Avoid use during the first and second trimester of pregnancy. Usage: oral, topical, inhalation. **Note:** Middle

Clary Sage can be used as a deodorant, antidepressant, and as a sedative. It is effective in combating oily hair and is a superior oil for acne, wrinkles and fine lines. Women experiencing hormonal changes or menopause symptoms such as hot flashes find this oil quite beneficial. Clary sage's properties are antidepressant, anticonvulsive, antispasmodic, anti-inflammatory, antiseptic, aphrodisiac, astringent, bactericidal, carminative, deodorant, digestive, emmenagogue, euphoric, hypotensive, nervine, sedative, stomachic, uterine and nerve tonic. Clary sage oil is non-toxic and non-sensitizing. Its anti-inflammatory and antispasmodic properties help to calm and soothe the body and mind. It also aids in reducing pain associated with inflammation. Do not use during pregnancy or if you are at risk for breast cancer as it may have an estrogen-like effect on the body. Usage: oral, topical, inhalation. **Note:** Top-Middle

Clove Bud has a spicy, rich scent and is an effective agent for minor aches and pains. Eugenol, the main compound in clove bud blocks the action of multiple inflammatory molecules involved in arthritis. Clove bud has antiseptic properties that can be used for acne, cuts and bruises, preventing infections and works as a pain reliever. It helps with toothaches, mouth sores, rheumatism, and arthritis. For the digestive system, it helps to prevent vomiting, diarrhea, flatulence, spasms, and parasites, as well as bad breath. Clove oil is valuable for relieving respiratory problems, like bronchitis, asthma, and tuberculosis. Its disinfecting feature makes it useful with infectious diseases. Clove oil's therapeutic properties are analgesic, antiseptic, antispasmodic, antineuralgic, anti-inflammatory, carminative, anti-infectious, disinfectant, insecticide, tonic, stomachic, rubefacient, uterine, and as a stimulant. Clove helps to reduce pain caused by inflammation and joint and muscle trauma. It increases blood flow and circulation throughout the body. This oil may cause sensitization in some individuals and should be used in dilution. Avoid use during pregnancy. Usage: oral, topical, inhalation. **Note:** Middle

Cilantro or Coriander works as an analgesic, antirheumatic, antispasmodic, carminative, deodorant, fungicidal and is revitalizing and stimulating. It relieves mental fatigue, migraine pain, stress, and nervous debility. Coriander's warming effect is helpful for alleviating pain such as rheumatism, arthritis and muscle spasms. It contains antibacterial compounds preventing salmonella, as well as possessing antimicrobial properties. The healing properties of cilantro or coriander oil are attributed to phytonutrient content, including carvone, geraniol, limonene, borneol, camphor, elemol, and linalool. Its active phenolic acid compounds, including caffeine and chlorogenic acid. Coriander has traditionally been referred to as an "anti-diabetic" herb and traditionally used in India for its anti-inflammatory properties. Recent studies conducted in the United States confirm Coriander's ability to reduce the number of damaged fats (lipid peroxides) in cells, lower cholesterol levels of total and LDL, and increase levels of HDL. Coriander oil is also beneficial for removing heavy metals and toxins from the body. Usage: topical, diffusion/inhalation, internal. **Note:** Top

Cypress is used for preventing excessive perspiration, particularly in the feet. It is suitable for hemorrhoids, oily skin and acts as an astringent in skin care applications. It is incredibly gentle and ideal for all skin types. This oil calms and soothes anger while having a positive effect on one's mood. It is suitable for various female problems and good for coughs and bronchitis. Cypress assists with varicose veins and bodily fluids by improving circulation. Its properties include antibacterial, anti-infectious, anti-inflammatory, antirheumatic, antiseptic, antispasmodic, astringent, decongestant, diuretic, and as a vein tonic. Avoid use during pregnancy. May interact with aspirin, blood pressure, antiplatelet, and anticoagulant medications. Usage: oral, topical, inhalation. **Note:** Middle-Base

Eucalyptus is perfect for sore muscles and joints since it helps to cool the affected area. Its health benefits attributed to as being anti-inflammatory, antispasmodic, antirheumatic, decongestant, deodorant, antiseptic, antibacterial, and stimulating. Eucalyptus helps to ease the pain while reducing inflammation. Its strong antibacterial properties assist with reducing inflammation due to infection. Do not ingest as this oil is considered toxic if taken internally. It is non-irritant and non-sensitive. Avoid use with epilepsy and Parkinson's disease. Do not use on children under five. It should be used in dilution. May interact with aspirin, blood pressure, antiplatelet, and anticoagulant medications and could increase the risk of bleeding among individuals with bleeding disorders. Please check with your healthcare provider before use during pregnancy. Usage: topical, inhalation. **Note:** Top

Fennel (Sweet) is credited with being carminative, depurative, diuretic, expectorant, laxative, and a stimulant. It is believed to be invigorating, restoring, stimulating, and warming. Fennel is credited as helping to promote healing of wounds or infections in the body, reducing inflammation. Because of its antispasmodic properties, fennel helps reduce pain. Its therapeutic properties include aperitif, antiseptic, antispasmodic, emmenagogue, galactagogue, stomachic, splenic, tonic, and vermifuge. Fennel is a stimulant which increased blood flow and circulation throughout the body. This oil may cause photosensitivity and contact dermatitis. Dilute well before use. Avoid use during pregnancy. Avoid use if you have epilepsy or Parkinson's disease. May interfere with the enzymes responsible for drug metabolism (NSAIDs, proton-pump inhibitors, acetaminophen, antiepileptics, antidepressants, antipsychotics, diabetic medications, antihistamines, antibiotics, and anesthetics). Use extremely diluted with children under six. Usage: topical. **Note:** Top-Middle

Frankincense is highly prized in the aromatherapy industry as a powerful anti-inflammatory with sedative properties. It is frequently used in skin care products as it is considered a valuable ingredient with remarkable anti-aging, rejuvenating and healing properties. Frankincense helps to reduce pain associated with inflammation, while calming the body and mind, promoting healing. It prevents infections with its antiseptic qualities. The therapeutic properties of frankincense oil are antiseptic, astringent, antirheumatic, antispasmodic, carminative, cicatrizant, cytophylactic, digestive, diuretic, emmenagogue, expectorant, sedative, tonic, uterine and vulnerary. Medical studies conducted on the use of frankincense boswellia in treating RA symptoms have shown positive results in reducing inflammation, pain, and stiffness. According to the Arthritis Foundation, the boswellic acids in frankincense extracts contain anti-inflammatory and analgesic properties that may help autoimmune responses and prevent cartilage damage May interfere with the enzymes responsible for drug metabolism (NSAIDs, proton-pump inhibitors, acetaminophen, antiepileptics, antidepressants, antipsychotics, diabetic medications, antihistamines, antibiotics, and anesthetics). Frankincense is non-toxic, non-irritant and non-sensitizing. Frankincense can be inhaled, applied topically, or ingested. Usage: oral, topical, inhalation. **Note:** Base

Galbanum is used externally as a poultice for inflammatory swelling, skin disorders, treating wounds, and for wounds that are slow in healing. It is known for its respiratory treatment for asthma, bronchitis, and chronic coughs. It is also good for digestive issues, panic attacks and conditions of claustrophobia. This oil's properties include analgesic, anti-arthritic, antirheumatic, antibacterial, antiviral, anti-inflammatory, antioxidant, antispasmodic, and as an immunostimulant. It aids circulation and the immune function. Galbanum is non-toxic, non-irritant and non-sensitizing. Usage: topical. **Note:** Top

Ginger is excellent for colds and flu, nausea (including motion sickness and morning sickness), rheumatism, coughs and circulation issues. It has warming properties that help to relieve muscular cramps, spasms, aches and eases stiffness in joints. It reduces inflammation and pain associated with headaches, colds, muscle strains, and arthritis. Ginger's healing properties include analgesic, anti-inflammatory, antiseptic, antispasmodic, rubefacient, carminative, tonic, diaphoretic, expectorant, and antiemetic. Humulene and zingiberene, two properties abundant in ginger, have been found to have anti-inflammatory, analgesic, anti-tumor, and anxiety-releasing properties. Research has been shown constituents in ginger decrease pain associated with arthritis by intercepting the vanilloid receptors, located on the sensory nerve endings, affecting the pain pathways and relieving inflammation and pain immediately. It may irritate sensitive skin. May interact with aspirin, blood pressure, antiplatelet, and anticoagulant medications. Usage: oral, topical, inhalation. **Note:** Base

Helichrysum is an effective oil for relieving pain and inflammation caused by arthritis. It is also aids in healing bruises, boils, burns, cuts, dermatitis, eczema, irritated skin, and wounds. It supports the body through post-viral fatigue and convalescence, and can also be used to repair skin damaged by psoriasis or ulceration. Helichrysum's therapeutic properties include anti-inflammatory, antibacterial, analgesic, antiseptic, antispasmodic, antifungal, antiviral, antimicrobial, and as a tonic for the nervous system. It is a great addition to a blend for muscle spasms. Helps to strengthen the circulatory system and clear blood clots. Research revealed helichrysum inhibited 5-LOX activity (a proinflammatory enzyme) and corticoid steroid-like properties in vitro. This oil is non-toxic, non-irritating and non-sensitizing. Please check with your healthcare provider before using during pregnancy. Usage: oral, topical, inhalation. **Note:** Base

Hyssop is known for its antirheumatic, antiseptic, antispasmodic, carminative, diuretic, sedative, stimulant, tonic and vulnerary agent properties. Historically, hyssop was referred to in the Bible for its cleansing action in connection with plague, leprosy and chest ailments. It has been used for purification and to ward off lice. Hyssop oil is non-irritant and non-sensitizing but does contain pinocamphone and should be used in moderation. Avoid use during pregnancy and by people with epilepsy. Usage: topical, inhalation. **Note:** Middle-Top

Juniper Berry is a supportive, restoring, and tonic aid. It is used in acne treatments, for oily skin, dermatitis, weeping eczema, psoriasis, and blocked pores. It is considered purifying and clearing. Juniper berry's therapeutic properties are antiseptic, anti-arthritic, antirheumatic, antispasmodic, astringent, carminative, depurative, diuretic, rubefacient, stimulating, stomachic, sudorific, and vulnerary. It clears the body of uric acid and returns skin tissue to normal functioning. Juniper is known to remove toxins from the body and increase blood flow allowing the white blood cells to reach the affected area quicker and promote healing. Its antispasmodic properties help to calm and relax injured muscles and reduce inflammation. Juniper Berry is non-irritating and non-sensitizing. May interact with diabetic medications and promote low blood sugar. Usage: oral, topical, inhalation. **Note:** Middle

Lavender has analgesic properties that ease the pain of a burn and prevents infection. Lavender also has cytophylactic properties that promote rapid healing and reduces scarring. Lavender does an excellent job at balancing oil production in the skin as well as clearing blemishes and evening skin tone and even helps to hydrate dry skin. Lavender is indicated for all skin types and can be used at any step in your skin care regimen. Lavender is beneficial for colds, flu, asthma, high blood pressure, and migraines. It is also excellent for helping with insomnia. The therapeutic properties of lavender oil are antiseptic, analgesic, anticonvulsant, antidepressant, antirheumatic, antispasmodic, anti-inflammatory, antiviral, bactericide, carminative, cholagogue, cicatrisant, cordial, cytophylactic, decongestant, deodorant, diuretic, emmenagogue, hypotensive, nervine, rubefacient, sedative, sudorific and vulnerary. Its anti-inflammatory properties help to reduce pain and inflammation in the affected area, promoting healing. In a study conducted in 2016, participants reported reduced pain who used a 5% diluted blend containing lavender and almond oil on their swollen joints (osteoarthritis) during the three-week study. Lavender is non-toxic, non-irritating and non-sensitizing. Do not use during the first trimester of pregnancy. Usage: oral, topical, inhalation. **Note:** Middle

Lavandin properties include analgesic, anticonvulsive, antidepressant, antiphlogistic, antirheumatic, antiseptic, antispasmodic, antiviral, bactericidal, carminative, cholagogue, cicatrizant, cordial, cytophylactic, decongestant, deodorant, and diuretic. It is considered one of the most useful and versatile essential oils from easing sore muscles and joints, relieving muscle stiffness, clearing the lungs and sinuses from phlegm to healing wounds and dermatitis. Lavandin is advantageous for burns and healing of the skin. Its antiseptic and analgesic properties aids with easing pain and preventing infection. Lavandin cytophylactic properties promote rapid healing and help reduce scarring. Its calming scent reduces anxiety and promotes sleep. This oil is non-toxic, non-irritating and non-sensitizing. Use caution during pregnancy. Usage: topical, inhalation. **Note:** Middle

Lemongrass is known for its stimulating qualities and makes an excellent antidepressant. Lemongrass enhances connective tissue repair. This essential oil is known to promote blood circulation by dilating the blood vessels, allowing uninterrupted blood flow. Lemongrass helps reduce inflammation. It has potent analgesic and anti-inflammatory properties. Lemongrass not only tones but fortifies the nervous system and can be used in the bath for soothing muscular nerves and pain with its potent analgesic and anti-inflammatory qualities. Lemongrass has an outstanding reputation for keeping insects away, controlling perspiration and for treating athlete's' foot. This oil relieves the symptoms of jet lag, helps with nervousness and anxiety, and clears headaches. It is useful for respiratory conditions such as sore throats, laryngitis and fever and helps prevent spreading of infectious diseases when diffused. It is also good for colitis, indigestion, and gastroenteritis. The therapeutic properties of lemongrass oil are analgesic, antidepressant, antimicrobial, antipyretic, antiseptic, astringent, bactericidal, carminative, deodorant, diuretic, febrifuge, fungicidal, galactagogue, insecticidal, nervine, nervous system sedative and tonic. This oil reduces inflammation by inhibiting the production of the proinflammatory cytokines (IL-1beta and IL-6). Citral is known to suppress the COX-2 enzyme (an enzyme present in cells when inflammation occurs in arthritis). Avoid use with individuals with glaucoma. Use caution in prostatic hyperplasia and with skin hypersensitivity or damaged skin. Avoid use during the first trimester of pregnancy. Avoid if you have a history of high blood pressure. Safe for topical and ingestion if diluted properly. A suggested safe limit for humans (based on an experiment in rats) is 0.7 mg/kg/day of the essential oil. Usage: oral, topical, inhalation. **Note:** Top

Lime has a crisp, refreshing citrus scent with uplifting and revitalizing properties that help with depression. It acts as an astringent on the skin and helps clear oily skin. Lime cools fevers due to colds and flu, eases coughs and strengthens the immune system as well as treats bronchitis, asthma, and sinusitis. Lime oil is also helpful for arthritis, rheumatism, poor circulation, and in eliminating cellulite and obesity. The therapeutic properties of lime are antiseptic, antiviral, astringent, aperitif, bactericidal, disinfectant, febrifuge, hemostatic, restorative and tonic. May interfere with enzymes responsible for metabolizing medications (NSAIDs, proton-pump inhibitors, acetaminophen, antiepileptics, immune modulators, blood-sugar medications, blood pressure medications, antidepressants, antipsychotics, diabetic medications, antihistamines, antibiotics, and anesthetics). Lime is considered phototoxic; users should avoid direct sunlight after application. Usage: oral, topical, inhalation. **Note:** Top

Marjoram is a comforting oil that can be massaged into the affected area or added to a warm compress to ease discomfort. It is useful for treating tired, aching muscles or in a sports massage blend. Marjoram's pain-relieving properties are helpful for rheumatic pains, sprains, spasms, as well as swollen joints and achy muscles. It can be added to a warm or hot bath for joint and muscle stiffness which can occur with arthritis. This oil is helpful for asthma and other respiratory complaints and has a calming effect on emotions, especially for hyperactive people. It soothes the digestive system and helps with indigestion, constipation, and flatulence. Marjoram is superb as a relaxant and is useful for headaches, migraines, and insomnia. Marjoram's therapeutic properties are analgesic, antispasmodic, anti-arthritic, antirheumatic, anaphrodisiac, antiseptic, antiviral, anti-inflammatory, bactericidal, carminative, cephalic, cordial, diaphoretic, digestive, diuretic, emmenagogue, expectorant, fungicidal, hypotensive, laxative, nervine, sedative, stomachic, vasodilator, and vulnerary. Its sedative properties allow the body to heal, reduce inflammation and eliminate pain. Marjoram is generally non-toxic, non-irritating and non-sensitizing. Usage: oral, topical, inhalation. **Note:** Middle

Myrrh is characterized as antimicrobial, antifungal, astringent, healing, tonic, stimulant, carminative, expectorant, diaphoretic, locally antiseptic, immune stimulant, bitter, circulatory stimulant, anti-inflammatory, and antispasmodic. Myrrh also helps with ailments such as colds, coughs, sore throats and bronchitis. Due to its antirheumatic, analgesic and anti-inflammatory properties, this oil is used to treat RA symptoms in alleviating joint pain and stiffness. Myrrh is used for diarrhea, dyspepsia, flatulence and hemorrhoids. It is commonly used for the treatment of mouth and gum infections, ulcers, gingivitis, and pyorrhea and is also good for skin infections such as boils, skin ulcers, bedsores, ringworm, wounds that won't heal, eczema and athlete's foot. Myrrh helps decrease inflammation by inhibiting the 5-lipoxygenase (5-LOX) enzyme that causes the inflammation response. Myrrh should be used in small amounts as it is considered possibly toxic in high concentrations and potentially harmful. Amounts larger than 2-4 grams can cause kidney complications and heart rate changes. Myrrh should not be used during pregnancy as it may stimulate the uterus and cause a miscarriage. Use during lactation is not recommended. Usage: oral, topical, inhalation. **Note:** Base

Patchouli is beneficial for combating nervous disorders, nausea, treats depression, and fever. This oil's therapeutic properties include antidepressant, anti-inflammatory, antimicrobial, antiseptic, antitoxic, antiviral, aphrodisiac, astringent, bactericidal, deodorant, diuretic, fungicidal, nervine, prophylactic, stimulating and tonic agent. Patchouli has been shown to stimulate cell regeneration. It is superb for mature, dry, and chapped skin. As a sedative oil, it allows the body to relax and rest, allowing healing to begin. In aromatherapy, it is an excellent fixative that can help extend other, more expensive oils. May interact with aspirin, blood pressure, antiplatelet, and anticoagulant medications, and increase the risk of bleeding among people with bleeding disorders. Usage: oral, topical, inhalation. **Note:** Base

Peppermint has long been credited as being useful in combating stomach ailments and soothing the digestive system. Great for headaches, travel sickness, and jet lag. It is viewed as an antispasmodic and antimicrobial agent. Most people know it as a flavoring or scenting agent in food and beverages. It is also a favorite for skin and hair care products (where it has a cooling effect by constricting capillaries and helps with bruises and sore joints). Peppermint's anti-inflammatory and pain-relieving properties help to reduce pain and swelling, as well as stiffness. Peppermint has been studied for its ability to kill pain by blocking substance P and calcium channels. In vitro peppermint showed to be a good free radical scavenger and significantly decreased uric acid levels in the blood (gout). Its properties include antifungal, antiseptic, antispasmodic, astringent, anti-inflammatory, analgesic, carminative, febrifuge, decongestant, expectorant, and stimulating to the circulatory and immune systems. Peppermint can be sensitizing due to the menthol content. Do not use if you have cardiac fibrillation. Avoid in children under six, as it may cause breathing problems. Use caution if you have high blood pressure. Usage: oral, topical, inhalation. **Note:** Top-Middle

Rose is an uplifting aphrodisiac and is wonderful for meditation. This oil is particularly beneficial for mature, dry, or sensitive skin. As a tonic, it has a soothing quality for inflammation and constricting action on capillaries. Rose oil is used in the treatment for depression, grief, anger, and other unpleasant emotions. It supports the heart and digestive systems and is considered one of the most incredible remedies for female problems such as balancing hormones during menopause. It helps to reduce muscle spasms and pain from injury and inflammation. The therapeutic properties of rose are antidepressant, antiphlogistic, antiseptic, antispasmodic, antiviral, aphrodisiac, astringent, bactericidal, choleretic, cicatrisant, depurative, emmenagogue, hemostatic, hepatic, laxative, nervous system sedative, stomachic and a tonic for the heart, liver, stomach, and uterus. Rose oil relieves pain by activating the TRPV1 receptor (a sensor that detects pain). Avoid use during the first trimester of pregnancy. Usage: oral, topical, inhalation. **Note:** Base

Rosemary stimulates cell renewal and improves dry or mature skin, eases lines and wrinkles, and heals burns and wounds. This warming oil improves circulation and can reduce the appearance of broken capillaries and varicose veins. Rosemary helps with overcoming mental fatigue and sluggishness by stimulating and strengthening the entire nervous system. It also enhances mental clarity while aiding alertness and concentration. Rosemary aids in reducing inflammation by increasing blood flow and circulation. This anti-inflammatory oil treats muscle pain as well as rheumatism by inhibiting the 5-lipoxygenase (5-LOX) enzyme that is involved in the inflammation response. It also reduces pain associated with inflammation. Rosemary is beneficial to use in stressful conditions. Rosemary is generally non-toxic and non-sensitizing but is not suitable for people with epilepsy or high blood pressure. Rosemary's therapeutic properties are analgesic, anti-inflammatory, antirheumatic, antiseptic, astringent, antispasmodic, antiviral, decongestant, diuretic, expectorant, restorative, and stimulant. Use caution with use during pregnancy. Avoid with children under six and those with epilepsy and Parkinson's disease. May interfere with enzymes that metabolize medications (NSAIDs, proton-pump inhibitors, acetaminophen, antiepileptics, immune modulators, blood sugar, and blood pressure medications, antihistamines, antibiotics, and anesthetics). Usage: oral (caution), topical, inhalation. **Note:** Middle

Sandalwood is known to create an exotic, sensual mood with a reputation as an aphrodisiac. In aromatherapy, it has been used for years to reduce and relieve inflammation. Its antiseptic properties help to reduce and eliminate infection that causes inflammation. Sandalwood is used to reduce swelling and muscle spasms by inhibiting the 5-lipoxygenase (5-LOX) enzyme that is involved in the inflammation response. Its sedative effect allows the body to relax and heal. Sandalwood is used to help combat bronchitis, chapped and dry skin, mood disturbances, stress and stretch marks. It is said to have antimicrobial properties which make it effective in treating skin conditions such as acne, oily skin, and eczema. It is especially beneficial for dehydrated skin. Sandalwood has powerful antibacterial and antifungal agents which makes it beneficial for chest infections and urinary tract infections. Sandalwood's therapeutic properties are antiphlogistic, antiseptic, antispasmodic, astringent, carminative, diuretic, emollient, expectorant, sedative, and tonic. Sandalwood is considered non-toxic, non-irritant and non-sensitizing. Usage: oral, topical, inhalation. **Note:** Base

Scotch Pine is documented as an analgesic, antibacterial, antibiotic, antifungal, antiseptic, and antiviral oil. Aromatherapists praise its use for arthritis, muscular aches and pain, rheumatism, and neuralgia. Animal research shows that pine oil contains monoterpenes that may protect against osteoporosis by inhibiting osteoclast activity (cells that break down bone tissue to release minerals into the circulatory system). It is also effective for upper respiratory infections due to colds and acts as a decongestant, treats coughs, bronchitis, sinusitis, asthma, and laryngitis. Scotch pine also treats bladder infections and cystitis, catarrh and acts as a cholagogue and circulatory agent. For the skin, it has been applied to cuts, eczema, lice, psoriasis, ringworm, and scrapes. Scotch pine is non-toxic and non-irritant. However, it should be used with caution and diluted when used on the skin. Usage: oral, topical, inhalation. **Note:** Top

Spruce is used for the treatment of asthma, bronchitis, coughs, colds, flu, infection, muscle aches and pains, poor circulation, and respiratory weakness. Spruce is used in baths for tired muscles, room sprays, detergents, and in cough and cold preparations. It is a popular choice for arthritis and rheumatism with its powerful anti-inflammatory properties. Spruce's therapeutic properties include anti-inflammatory, antirheumatic, antispasmodic, antiseptic, decongestant, diuretic, rubefacient and warming. At low doses, it is non-toxic, non-irritating, and non-sensitizing. Usage: oral, topical, inhalation. **Note:** Middle

Thyme is considered a stimulating, uplifting, and reviving oil with antiseptic qualities. The therapeutic properties of Thyme oil are antirheumatic, antiseptic, antispasmodic, bactericidal, bechic, cardiac, carminative, cicatrizant, diuretic, emmenagogue, expectorant, hypertensive, insecticide, stimulant, tonic, and vermifuge. It helps with mental concentration and works well as a bronchial and lung tonic making it valuable for bronchitis, coughs, colds, and asthma. Thyme's warming qualities make it great for rheumatism, sciatica, arthritis, and gout. Red thyme and white thyme are both used in aromatherapy. It has anti-inflammatory and antispasmodic properties which help reduce and relieve inflammation in the body with its chemical component, carvacrol (alpha-terpineol CT). Thyme oil helps to increase blood flow and circulation which promotes healing as well as removes toxins from the body. Its antiseptic properties help to reduce and prevent infection. Thyme is a potential skin irritant. Avoid use during pregnancy and with epilepsy. Usage: oral (caution), topical, inhalation. **Note:** Middle-Top

Turmeric has been traditionally used as a favorite Asian and Middle Eastern spice in cooking for centuries. Its healing properties as a strong relaxant and balancer are due to a prominent active component called curcumin which has been found to help protect joints from inflammation. It has historical applications as an antiseptic aid for skin care and as an analgesic for painful joint conditions such as rheumatism. It helps decrease inflammation by actively inhibiting the 5-lipoxygenase (5-LOX) enzyme that is involved in inflammation. This oil makes an excellent digestive aid and helps to reduce excess fluid. Its therapeutic properties include analgesic, anti-inflammatory, carminative, tonic, and diuretic. Turmeric has potential irritating and toxic effects when used in large concentrations. May interact with aspirin, blood pressure, antiplatelet, diabetes medication, and anticoagulant medications. Usage: oral, topical, inhalation. **Note:** Base

Vetiver is profoundly relaxing and comforting. Its calming and soothing effect helps to relieve and reduce symptoms of inflammation. It helps to promote circulation and reduce pain. Its antiseptic properties can help to reduce infection and promote healing. This oil is useful in dispelling irritability, anger, and hysteria while having a balancing effect on the hormonal system. Vetiver helps to reduce wrinkles and stretch marks while nourishing and moisturizing the skin. It is also beneficial for helping wounds heal. Vetiver oil's therapeutic properties are antiseptic, aphrodisiac, cicatrizant, nervine, sedative, tonic, and vulnerary. There is no known toxicity. Usage: oral, topical, inhalation. **Note:** Base

Wintergreen serves as an anti-inflammatory, antiseptic, diuretic, stimulant, emmenagogue, and antirheumatic. It is beneficial in rheumatic conditions and helps with muscular pains and arthritis, especially for athletes. Wintergreen contains methyl salicylate which is similar to aspirin – a component that relieves pain often associated with inflammation. It also has antiseptic properties which help with reducing the inflammation caused by infection. It has stimulant properties which help in promoting and increasing blood flow and circulation to promote healing. Wintergreen has a cortisone-like effect that supports bone healing. Avoid use during pregnancy. Safety with nursing women or those with severe liver or kidney disease is not known. Wintergreen should be avoided by children under age 12 to prevent salicylate poisoning and serious adverse effects. Usage: topical (dilute for topical use), inhalation. **Note:** Middle

Yarrow is credited with having an energy similar to that of the earth. It is a balancing, uplifting oil with practical applications on gynecological issues, wounds, and open sores. This is an exceptional oil for reducing swelling, muscle spasms, digestive issues, indigestion, irritable bowel syndrome, and flatulence. It is also beneficial as an anti-inflammatory for muscle and joint conditions. Yarrow helps promote circulation and relieve inflammation commonly associated with arthritis. Its antispasmodic properties soothe and heal. The therapeutic properties of yarrow are analgesic, anti-allergenic, antidepressant, anti-inflammatory, antiseptic, antiviral, cicatrizant, decongestant, digestive aid, and diuretic. The intensity of this blue-green colored oil comes from it chamazulene content, which is a potent anti-inflammatory agent and is effective for nerve pains, muscle injuries, tendonitis, and arthritis. Yarrow has no known toxicity and is non-irritant in low concentration. Usage: oral, topical, inhalation. **Note:** Middle

THERAPEUTIC PROPERTIES

Analgesic: Balsam fir, basil, bay laurel, bergamot, birch, black pepper, blue cypress, blue spruce, blue tansy, cajeput, camphor, cassia, cinnamon, citronella, clove, copaiba, coriander, eucalyptus, fennel, frankincense, galbanum, geranium, German chamomile, ginger, helichrysum, juniper berry, lavandin, lavender, lemon, lemon verbena, lemongrass, marjoram, melaleuca (tea tree), neroli, niaouli, nutmeg, oregano, palo santo, peppermint, pine, ravensara, ravintsara, Roman chamomile, rosemary, sandalwood, silver fir, spearmint, spike lavender, spruce (black), thyme, tsuga, turmeric, vetiver, white fir, wintergreen

Anti-arthritic: Cassia, frankincense, galbanum, German chamomile, juniper berry, marjoram, ravintsara, rosemary, silver fir, thyme, turmeric, vetiver, white fir, wintergreen

Anti-inflammatory: Balsam fir, basil, bay laurel, bergamot, birch, black pepper, blue cypress, blue spruce, blue tansy camphor, cedarwood, cistus, citronella, clove, copaiba, cypress, frankincense, galbanum, geranium, German chamomile, ginger, goldenrod, helichrysum, lavender, lemon, lemon verbena, lemongrass, lime, marjoram, melaleuca (tea tree), myrrh, neroli, orange, oregano, palo santo, patchouli, petitgrain, pine, ravintsara, Roman chamomile, rose, sage, sandalwood, silver fir, spearmint, spike lavender, spikenard, spruce (black), tangerine, thyme, tsuga, turmeric, vetiver, white fir, wintergreen, ylang ylang

Antirheumatic: Balsam fir, bay laurel, camphor, cassia, cedarwood, citronella, coriander, eucalyptus, frankincense, galbanum, German chamomile, juniper berry, lemon, marjoram, niaouli, nutmeg, pine, ravintsara, Roman chamomile, rosemary, silver fir, thyme, turmeric, vetiver, white fir, wintergreen

Antispasmodic: Balsam fir, basil, bay laurel, bergamot, birch, blue tansy, cajeput, camphor, cardamom, cassia, cedarwood, citronella, clove, coriander, cypress, eucalyptus, galbanum, German chamomile, ginger, helichrysum, juniper berry, lavandin, lavender, lemon verbena, lime, marjoram, melissa, myrrh, neroli, niaouli, nutmeg, orange, oregano, palo santo, peppermint, petitgrain, ravensara, Roman chamomile, rose, rosemary, sage, sandalwood, silver fir, spearmint, spike lavender, spikenard, spruce (black), tangerine, thyme, turmeric, vetiver, white fir, wintergreen, ylang ylang

Bone Pain Relievers: Balsam fir, wintergreen

Bone Turnover, Promotes Healthy: Pine, rosemary, sage, thyme

Circulation Aids/Stimulants: Basil, birch, black pepper, cajeput, carrot seed, cassia, cedarwood, cinnamon, clove, coriander, cypress, galbanum, ginger, goldenrod, helichrysum, lemongrass, lime, marjoram, myrrh, niaouli, palmarosa, silver fir, white fir

Circulation/Redness, Increases Localized: Camphor, nutmeg, patchouli, rosemary, silver fir, spike lavender, spruce (black), thyme, tsuga, vetiver, white fir

Warming: Balsam fir, basil, bay laurel, cajeput, cardamom, coriander, cypress, marjoram, melissa, oregano, spruce (black), turmeric, wintergreen

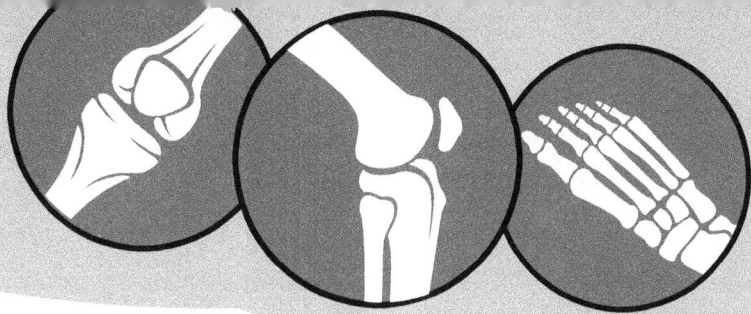

HOW TO USE ESSENTIAL OILS FOR ARTHRITIS

Incorporating essential oils and natural remedies such as aromatherapy and relaxation techniques into your life can be very beneficial for some health conditions. Most essential oils are safe and free of adverse side effects when used correctly. However, as with any substance you are introducing into your body, it is essential to use them intelligently.

While many people with arthritis can benefit from certain essential oils that contain terpenoid compounds such as linalool and 1,8 cineole that decrease inflammation, there are some factors you must consider:

Dosage – Dose is the most significant factor in essential oil usage. Some essential oils used in the wrong doses such as in too high of a concentration have been found (in animal and laboratory studies) to cause adverse effects in the body. Some essential oils can damage the skin, liver and other organs if misused.

Quality – The purity of the essential oil is important. Even when oil is labeled as pure, it may be adulterated with added synthetic chemicals, vegetable oil, or cheaper essential oils with similar scents. Make sure your oils are therapeutic quality.

Application – An essential oil that is safe when applied in one way may not be safe when used in another way. Some oils are considered safe if inhaled, and yet may be irritating if applied to the skin in concentration. For instance, citrus oils such as bergamot and lemon can cause phototoxicity (severe burn to the skin) if a person is exposed to the sun after topical application. However, this would not result from inhalation.

Lifestyle – Since arthritis is a debilitating health condition, it is important to combine your use of essential oils with diet and lifestyle changes to achieve success with your natural remedy.

Drug Interaction – If you're currently under a doctor's care for OA or RA, talk to your doctor before starting any treatment program with essential oils. You will want to make sure that your use of oils will not interfere with medications you are prescribed.

Another option is to find a naturopath to talk about holistic health care that looks at your health as a whole instead of treating symptoms of individual conditions. As you study and research therapeutic quality essential oils, you will find these are a great way to complement your whole body care, instead of taking a handful of pills every day for multiple medical issues.

SPECIAL NOTE:

Essential oils are not a "magic bullet." The suggestions for use of essential oils in this book are for you to use as complementary care to the healthcare plan you already have in place. It may be necessary for you to make changes in your diet and other lifestyle modifications for all things to work together. If you do not achieve satisfactory results in normalizing or managing your pain, please seek professional medical help.

WAYS TO USE ESSENTIAL OILS FOR ARTHRITIS

There are several options available for treating arthritis in both allopathic and alternative medicine. Many people today can manage their pain with the help of therapeutic quality essential oils along with vigilance and commitment to a healthy diet and lifestyle.

Various mechanisms can be used to deliver essential oils to target sites in the body. Typical routes of administration include topically, inhalation, and ingestion. Regardless of which route of administration is used, the essential oils have to travel to the site of action with either the help of blood, nerves or oxygen (when the inhalation route is used). Using a combination of these three approaches for reducing pain and relieving inflammation in the body will ensure success.

TIP: Individuals with RA may want to take frankincense capsules that contain at least 60 percent boswellic acid. Suggested dosage is 300–400 milligrams (mg) daily.

TOPICALLY

You can apply the essential oil(s) of choice to the affected area either on its own or mixed with a lotion or salve to apply to the affected area. Try combining a couple of oils to create a synergistic blend for multiple health benefits. When using an essential oil topically, be sure to dilute with a carrier oil. Essential oils are potent and direct application, or "neat," may cause irritation to the skin. Also, combining essential oils with a carrier base oil such as almond or coconut oil can add additional benefits as well for your arthritis treatment. Topically is one of the easiest and effective ways to use essential oils for arthritis. For example, massage stimulates circulation of the blood while reducing muscular tension, aches and pain, and inflammation. Also, it significantly reduces stress and can offer comfort and peace of mind, allowing healing to take place. Caution should be exercised when using any topical aromatherapy preparations around drug injection sites or areas of the body where transdermal medications are in use (i.e., estrogen or nicotine patches, etc.).

The absorption of certain essential oil chemical compounds has been confirmed through analysis of blood concentrations with maximum levels attained in as little as 10 minutes.

- **Roll On** – Use a rollerball applicator to apply an oil blend where needed. Reapply several times a day as needed.

- **Rub On** – Rub 1-2 drops of essential oil directly "neat" on the joint or affected area. Or, rub essential oil or essential oil blend on the bottom of feet each evening before bed.

- **Massage** – Massage an essential oil blend (with a carrier oil) for several minutes over the affected area. Reapply as desired.

ORALLY

You can try taking the essential oil or oils orally to help heal the inflammation inside the body. Be sure the essential oils you choose are **safe for ingestion**. Not all essential oils are safe for ingesting orally.

If you are considering ingesting essential oils, you will want to treat your essential oils like powerful medicines, because that is what they are. Taking an oil orally is nearly ten times stronger than when applied topically, so its smart to start with a tiny amount and increase gradually. While many essential oils are safe when used internally, some are not. Be sure to read about the oil and do your research to know of any warnings or contradictions. Also, you will want to be aware of proper dosage protocols. The necessary internal dose and frequency are dependent on several factors such as age, size, and health condition which will vary from person to person.

One essential oil company stated on their website, "The recommended internal dose of essential oils is 1–5 drops, depending on the oil or blend." Taking more than that is not advantageous; in fact, it can be harmful. It is better to take a smaller dose, which can be repeated every 4–6 hours as needed. A low daily dose is recommended for extended internal use.

Ingestion of certain essential oils may not serve to be the most efficient method for absorption into the bloodstream. They are absorbed into systemic circulation via the digestive tract. However, when taken orally, essential oils may lose some of the active principal compounds due to the first pass hepatic metabolism.

There are several methods for taking essential oils. In this book, internal use will comprise of consuming essential oils by mouth in a vegetable capsule, or by adding oil to honey, or on a sugar cube. Essential oils taken by mouth not in a capsule may be absorbed through the cheeks, the tongue or the lining of the throat. Essential oils are highly concentrated and potent – treat them like you would with any other highly concentrated pharmaceutical. It is recommended when using essential oils internally to seek the advice of a certified medical practitioner who is also trained in aromatherapy or a certified aromatherapist who is also trained in internal ingestion for the best protocol.

When using essential oils internally, use doses in the range of one to three drops, one to two times a day (for adults) and follow a protocol appropriate for your health. Store your oils in a safe place away from children. Using the appropriate amount of essential oil in a vegetable capsule that has been properly diluted will ensure it is maximally absorbed by the gut for the whole body effect. But like medicines, essential oil ingestion carries with it the potential for side effects, mild to severe, including seizures and poisoning.

- **Capsules** – Add one or two drops of essential oil to a "00" gelatin capsule filled with a carrier oil such as olive or coconut oil to buffer the essential oil. Take orally as you would with traditional supplements. A single oil or essential oil blend may be used in this way. For example, a capsule can be filled with 20% essential oil diluted with 80% vegetable oil (one ml=20 drops approximately). Each "00" capsule holds approximately 0.7-.91mL or 14 drops, and "0" capsules hold ten drops of oil. Enteric-coated gelatin capsules could be used as well since they do not release the essential oil until they are in the small intestine.

- **Juice or Water** – Add one or two drops of essential oil to a small glass of juice. Stir to blend well as oil will tend to float on the surface. A solubol can be added as a dispersant to distribute the oils.

- **Tea** – Add one or two drops of essential oil to a teaspoon of honey and stir into a cup of tea or warm water. Be sure not to overheat the water, as oils will evaporate. Sip slowly.

- **Swishing** – Add several drops of essential oil to a cup of water and swish around the mouth before swallowing.

- **Sugar Cube** – Use a dropper to add one or two drops of essential oil to a cube of sugar. It can be taken directly or added to a drink.

- **Honey** – Essential oils can be blended with honey water. Mix 1-2 drops essential oil into 1 Tsp. honey, add warm water and drink. Or add 1-2 drops of essential oil or essential oil blend to a tablespoon of honey, stir with a toothpick, and take orally.

For adults, the recommended oral dosage with essential oils is 1-3 drops, two to three times a day. The maximum daily dose is 12 drops. Some essential oil websites recommend up to 20 drops a day, which is quite high and is therefore not recommended. Some professionals recommend using essential oils two weeks out of the month or taking one drop, three times a day for an extended period. Others suggest using 1-2 drops, two to three times a day for five days and take two days rest. Either way, it is advisable to take breaks in your essential oil usage.

INHALATION

Try putting your essential oil or oils of choice in a diffuser to help relieve inflammation in the body. Inhaling can be very helpful when trying to reduce inflammation associated with headaches or respiratory problems such as asthma. Inhalation of certain essential oil's vapors triggers the olfactory bulb, which immediately sends a neurochemical signal to neuro-receptors. For example, smelling lavender essential oil triggers the release of serotonin from the raphe nucleus in the brain and produces a calmative effect. Essential oils can easily be absorbed via inhalation and enter the bloodstream to deliver healing constituents throughout the body. Inhalation presents the least amount of risk with most individuals.

- **Diffuse** – Use a nebulizer to diffuse your choice of oils for an hour, three times a day. You may want to use one specific essential oil (with no carrier oil added). Or, you may blend a combination of essential oils.

- **Cup Hands** – Place 2-3 drops of your chosen essential oil in your hand and rub your palms together. Cup hands over your nose and inhale deeply.

- **Inhaler** – Add 1-2 drops of essential oil to a tissue and carry with you to smell throughout the day or add several drops of pure essential oil to a pocket diffuser and use 2-3 times daily.

MASSAGE

Treat yourself to a massage to relieve extreme stress. Arthritic patients have found that massage therapy and gentle stretching helps to relieve pain, relax muscles, reduce swelling and aid in a range of motion in joints. A massage also boosts the blood flow to the impacted location, which helps to improve lymph drainage and warms the area being massaged. The rubbing will also drive the oils deeper, increasing absorption.

If you are unable to afford a massage, check online for more information on how to do a self-massage or watch a video for instructions on how to give yourself a massage. Here are some basic guidelines.

For osteoarthritis: Gently massage around the painful area with massage oil on your fingertips, making small, gentle circles with your fingertips. Avoid massaging directly on the joint. Instead, work right above and below it with your fingertips. Repeat daily for three to five minutes each time.

For rheumatoid arthritis: Apply oil or cream to your fingers and use a rhythmic or effleurage massage on the muscle and tissue around the afflicted joint. Repeat daily for five to ten minutes each time.

TIP: A general rule of thumb when diluting essential oils is to use one ounce of carrier oil for every 12 drops of essential oil.

HOW LONG SHOULD I USE ESSENTIAL OILS?

It is recommended to continue essential oil therapy for a few days or more following relief of symptoms to ensure complete healing occurs. A general rule of thumb in aromatherapy is that for every year you have suffered from a chronic condition, it could take one month of therapy to correct the condition. For acute conditions, if you do not obtain results within an hour or so, try a different essential oil or method of application. Keep in mind, everyone responds differently, and you may need to use more or less essential oil, depending on how your body reacts.

BUILDING UP A TOLERANCE TO ESSENTIAL OILS

It is safe to use the recipes in this book as recommended several times a day for a week or more. However, most aromatherapists recommend limiting the use of the same oil or essential oil blend to 21 days before taking a week break. It is suggested after regularly continued use to rotate your blends and use different oils or blends.

ROTATE YOUR OILS

After regularly continued use of the same oil or blend, you should rotate your blends and use different oils. This is recommended for two reasons. First, this reduces to the possibility of a risk of sensitization to the essential oil or blend that you are using. In rare cases, the immune system could be triggered by having an inflammatory skin reaction, respiratory problem or anaphylactic shock.

Secondly, this also reduces the chance of your body developing a resistance or becoming acclimated to the effectiveness of the essential oils you are using. In other words, the essential oil blend may no longer work or provide the same positive benefits it once did.

TIP: If you start to have any unusual side effects, discontinue use immediately and talk to your doctor. They will help you determine the cause and assist you in following the best arthritis management plan.

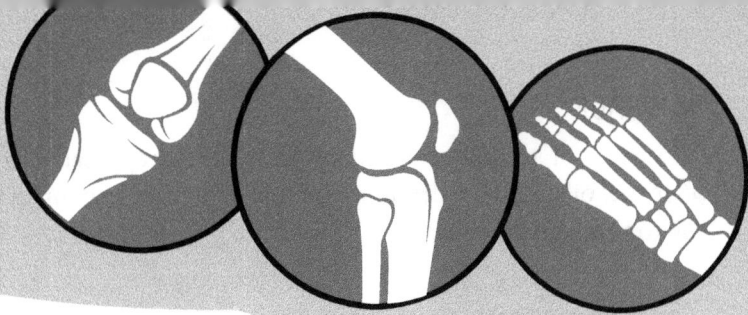

OTHER METHODS OF USE

BATH

For a full bath, mix 8-10 drops of essential oil into two ounces of sea salts or a cup of milk then pour into a running bath. Agitate water in a figure-eight motion to make sure the oil is mixed well, preventing irritation to mucous membranes. Another method is to add essential oils after the bath has been drawn. Mix essential oils into a palm full of liquid soap, shampoo or a tablespoon of Jojoba oil and swish around to dissolve in the tub. Soak for 15-20 minutes.

SHOWER

While showering, add a drop or two of essential oil to a washcloth and rub on the body.

MASSAGE

A variety of techniques used in massage therapy can incorporate the use of essential oils. Add 6-9 drops of essential oil to 1 tablespoon of your favorite carrier oil to massage into body.

LOTIONS/CREAMS

Blending essential oils in an unscented, natural lotion/cream base allow you to benefit from the therapeutic qualities of the essential oil, giving you a non-oily way to apply essential oils. This is especially useful for someone with a skin condition that does not do well with oils. The dilution rate for using essential oils in a lotion base is no more than 2%. For adults, use 20 drops of essential oil to four ounces of lotion. For children and the elderly, use ten drops of essential oil to four ounces of lotion.

BODY OILS

Mix 30 drops of essential oil per one ounce of cold-pressed carrier oil such as coconut oil. Choose an all-purpose oil that relieves stress and/or tension, headaches, and smells terrific.

INHALATION

Inhalation can be enhanced with the use of a nebulizer or a cool-mist diffuser in which essential oils are dispersed into the air. Other devices such as a light ring, vaporizer, or electric burner may be used instead, though heating oils may alter their molecular structure and cause loss of some of their effectiveness. Inhalation is one of the most natural methods of use and is considered the most direct pathway for an aromatic blend or essence. When inhaled, fragrant vapors enter the lungs and are instantly released into the bloodstream for delivery to every cell in the body. Scientific research shows that essential oils can remain in a person's bloodstream for up to 4-6 hours, depending on the essential oil.

Essential oils that are properly diffused are known to kill bacteria and viruses, improve mental clarity, enhance or calm emotions, and increase feelings of well-being. Over time, oils diffused can strengthen the immune system, reduce mold, and eliminate unpleasant odors. If a diffuser is not available, making a room spray, personal inhaler, or placing a few drops on a tissue to inhale will suffice. All are very effective ways to benefit from the healing properties of essential oils. For inhalation, use intermittent exposure (not more than 15 minutes in an hour).

DIRECT INHALATION

Apply 2-3 drops of essential oils into your hand and rub palms together. Cup hands over the nose and mouth. Inhale vapors deeply several times.

HUMIDIFIER/VAPORIZER

For a humidifier or vaporizer, place 10 drops of essential oil undiluted into the unit.

NEBULIZER/DIFFUSER

Place 25 drops of essential oil undiluted inside the diffuser and use as needed. Limit diffusion of new oils to 10 minutes each day increasing the time until the desired effects are reached. Adjust times for different-sized rooms and the strength of each fragrance. Unlike cheap fragrant oils purchased at department stores to mask odors, diffusing pure essential oils alters the structure of the molecules that create odors – rendering them harmless. Essential oils increase the available oxygen in the room and produce negative ions, which kill microbes.

TIPS

- Sea salt baths are great to use when treating arthritis. They stimulate natural circulation and when used in high concentration help relieve arthritis symptoms. Sea salts and Epsom salts are great to use in baths for help ease the pain.

- For joint stiffness, try blending rosemary and lemongrass essential oils. They can help remove lactic acid buildup in the muscles, which attributes to causing stiffness. Add one drop each to 1/2 teaspoon carrier oil and massage into affected areas. Another great oil as a substitute is helichrysum italicum.

- Cold or warm compresses can be used in conjunction with any of the recipes. Whenever you apply heat or cold to the affected joints, be sure to move them as much as possible immediately afterward. Otherwise, it will defeat the purpose of the treatment.

- Massage and therapeutic baths will be your best methods of treatment. They will stimulate the circulation and help get rid of toxins and absorb minerals needed to function correctly. Gently massage muscles surrounding painful joints.

- An infusion of **St. John's Wort** is the best carrier oil for pain relief as it has natural analgesic properties of its own.

- Everyone is unique and what works for your condition may not work as well for another. Be willing to try different combinations to find which recipe helps you the most.

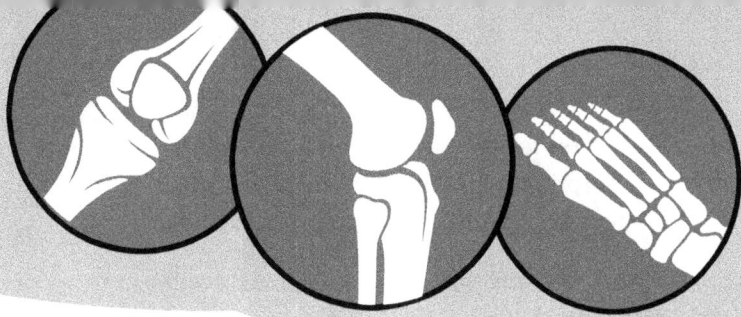

ESSENTIAL OIL SAFETY

In general, essential oils are safe to use for aromatherapy and therapeutic purposes. Nevertheless, safety must be exercised due to their potency and high concentration. Please read and follow these guidelines to obtain the maximum effectiveness and benefits.

- Avoid sunbathing, tanning booths, or saunas immediately after using essential oils.

- Be careful to avoid getting essential oils in the eyes. If you do splash a drop or two of essential oil in the eyes, use a small amount of olive oil (or another carrier oil) to dilute the essential oil and absorb with a washcloth. If severe, seek medical attention immediately.

- Take extra precaution when using oils with children. Never use undiluted essential oils on babies and always store your essential oils out of the reach of children.

- Never take essential oils internally without knowledge of its effect or proper usage. Seek the advice of a knowledgeable medical practitioner or another qualified clinical aromatherapist.

- If a dangerous quantity of essential oil has been ingested, immediately drink olive oil and induce vomiting. The olive oil will help in slowing down its absorption and will dilute the essential oil. Do not drink water—this will speed up the absorption of the essential oil.

- Most essential oils should be diluted before applying topically. Pay attention to safety guidelines—certain essential oils, such as cinnamon and clove bud, may cause skin irritation for those with sensitive skin.

  If you experience slight redness or itchiness, put olive oil (or any carrier oil) on the affected area and cover with a soft cloth. The olive oil acts as an absorbent fat and binds to the oil, diluting its strength and allowing it to be immediately removed. Aloe Vera gel also works well as an alternative to olive oil. Never use water to dilute essential oil—this will cause it to spread and enlarge the affected area. Redness or irritation may last 20 minutes to an hour.

- Never use oils undiluted on your skin. Always dilute with a carrier oil. If redness, burning, itching, or irritation occurs, stop using oil immediately. Be sure to wash hands after handling pure, undiluted essential oils.

- For sensitive skin or when using a new oil, perform a "Skin Patch Test." If irritation occurs, discontinue use of such oil or blend. See section, Skin Patch Test.

- If you are pregnant, lactating, suffer from epilepsy, have cancer, liver damage, or another medical condition, use essential oils under the care and supervision of a qualified aromatherapist or medical practitioner.

- To prevent contact sensitization (redness or irritation of skin due to repeated use of same individual oil) use different oils.

- Rotating essential oils is the most efficient and safest way to use them. Choose one essential oil or blend and try it first for a couple of weeks (up to 21 days), then switch to another oil.

- Be sure to check with your doctor before using essential oils. Some prescription medications contraindicate the use of some essential oils. Never replace prescribed medication for RA with essential oils, unless advised by the doctor.

- Less is best when taking essential oils internally. Take fewer drops at one time every 4-6 hours, versus more at one time.

SKIN PATCH TEST

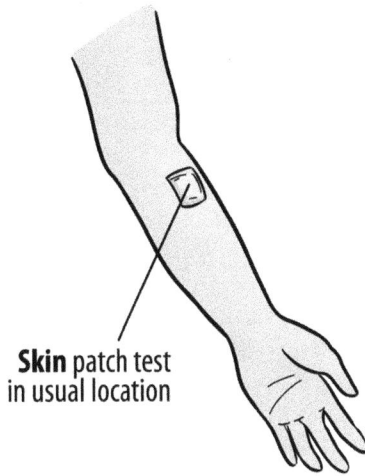

Skin patch test
in usual location

Certain essential oils can cause sensitization or an allergic reaction in some individuals. When using a new oil for the first time, you may want to perform a simple skin patch test on the inside of your arm or your chest. Place one drop of the essential oil into a carrier oil. Apply one drop on the skin and cover with a bandage. If the skin becomes irritated and red, remove the bandage and immediately wash the area with soap and water. If after 12 hours no irritation has occurred, it is safe to use on the skin.

For someone who tends to be highly allergic, here is a simple test to determine if he or she is sensitive to a particular carrier oil and essential oil.

1. First, rub a drop of carrier oil onto the upper chest. In 12 hours, check for redness or other skin irritation.

2. If the skin remains clear, place one drop of selected essential oil in 15 drops of the same carrier oil, and again rub into the upper chest. If no skin reaction appears after 12 hours, it is safe to use the carriers and the essential oil.

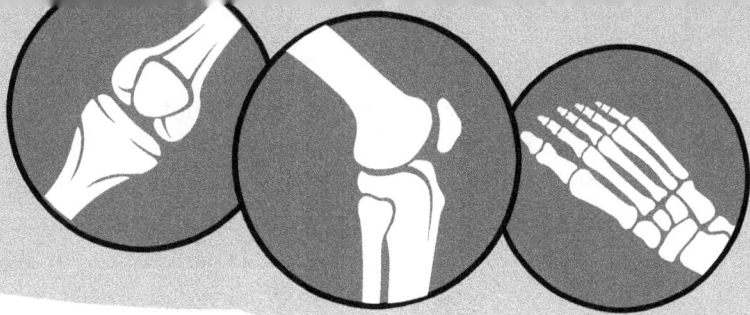

CARRIER OILS FOR ARTHRITIS BLENDS

When you use essential oils, in most cases you will want to dilute with a carrier or vegetable oil. Carrier oils come from nuts, seeds or kernels that contain essential fatty acids, fat-soluble vitamins, minerals, and other crucial nutrients. You will find a variety of carrier oils to choose from, each possessing different therapeutic properties.

The two primary methods of producing carrier oil are cold-pressed and maceration. These processes ensure they have not been modified by heat, which would destroy the vital nutrients contained in the oil and are as natural and unadulterated as possible.

Macerated oils, such as calendula and carrot oils, are made from a combination of a base oil such as sunflower and plant material that has been left in an airtight container over a period of time to infuse the liquid with the plant's constituents.

Carrier oils and infused oils are used to dilute essential oils and absolutes by offering the necessary lubrication and moisture to the skin for aromatherapy.

Distinct from essential oils, carrier oils do not contain aromatic scents (or only a very faint scent) and evaporate due to their large molecular structure. For this reason, most consider carrier oils just a vehicle for applying essential oils to the skin in massage. However, they do offer their healing properties which essential oils do not possess. Your aromatherapy experience can be significantly enhanced by choosing the best combination of carrier and essential oils. Sweet almond, fractionated coconut, avocado are excellent choices to use.

Carrier Oil	Shelf Life
Almond (sweet)	12 months
Apricot Kernel	6-12 months
Argan	24 months
Avocado	12 months
Borage	6 months
Carrot Seed	12 months
Cocoa Butter	3-5 years
Coconut (fractionated)	Indefinite
Coconut (virgin)	2-4 years
Evening Primrose	6-12 months
Grapeseed	3-6 months (up to 9 months, if refrigerated)
Hemp Seed	12 months
Jojoba	Indefinite
Olive	12-18 months
Safflower	24 months
Shea Butter	Indefinite
Walnut	12 months

TIP: A massage oil blend with a mixture of 10-15% essential oil and 85-90% carrier oil will ensure a powerful massage oil that is smooth and great-smelling.

SHELF LIFE OF CARRIER OILS

A carrier oil's shelf life, which is the length of time before a particular oil begins to turn rancid, can be significantly influenced by heat and light. You will want to store your oils in a cool, dark place to preserve their freshness, and in some cases refrigerate, as heat and sunlight can shorten their shelf life. When refrigerating, oils may appear cloudy but will regain their transparent state upon returning to room temperature. If you have a large amount of carrier oil on hand, you can freeze the unused portion until ready for use.

TIP: Try not to mix too much of your favorite massage blend in advance if you don't plan on using it right away.

Instead of thinking of carrier oils as merely the method of applying essential oils, explore the unique qualities of carrier oils separately to find the best oil for relieving pain and inflammation due to arthritis. You can enhance your benefits by using specific essential oils with carriers that increase their medicinal qualities. For this reason, consideration will be given to how plant-derived oils deliver health from the outside in. Externally applied oils help the body maintain vital functions in unique ways through both chemical changes and mechanical assistance.

Most carrier oils are unsaturated fats. Saturated fats have carbon bonds that do not bind to other carbon atoms. These oils are solid at room temperature and include animal-derived fats and some plant-derived fats as well. Coconut oil is a saturated fat that is often used as a carrier oil. Fractionated coconut, another common carrier oil, occurs when a coconut molecule has been altered to keep it in a liquid, rather than solid, state. The healing qualities of the oil are not compromised, and the oil can be used the same way a seed or nut oil is used.

When considering vegetable oils for use in capsules, many have the essential fatty acids Omega-6 (linoleic acid) and Omega-3 (linolenic). Essential fatty acids must be acquired through outside sources, primarily through diet, and are critical to maintaining health. According to aromatherapist Salvatore Battaglia, Omega-6, which is vital for skin, hair, liver function, joints, healing wounds, and circulation, is especially powerful in evening primrose oil, a popular and versatile carrier oil. Omega-3 is also in many carrier oils. Taken internally, it helps with vision, muscles, and growth. It is found in fish and some vegetable oils, like linseed and canola. It is known to boost circulation, assist in heart health, blood pressure and prevent inflammation. The most important thing to remember about lipid structure in carrier oils is that choosing high-quality, nutritious oils will significantly assist in their vital functions.

Carrier oils are primarily derived from nuts and seeds. They are extracted via cold-pressed technology, meaning high heat is not used. Once oils reach temperatures exceeding 160 degrees Celsius, their structure is altered, making them trans-fats, a kind of mutated fat that the body cannot assimilate properly. Expeller pressing is another common extraction method. By placing seeds or nuts in an expeller, the precious oil is pressed out and then bottled. Superior carrier oils are mechanically pressed oils and have not been subjected to chemical changes.

When carrier oils are used with essential oils topically, they provide a mechanism for the volatile oils to be transported more effectively. Most essential oils, when applied externally, move through the body system in an hour. A carrier oil, which is thicker than a volatile oil, "holds" the essential oil in place, delivering longer-lasting healing. You want to include the specific healing benefits of carrier oils in your aromatherapy applications as well; it might be useful to look at how carrier oils are sometimes categorized.

Essential oils in aromatherapy are highly concentrated and potent. Although there are only a few exceptions to using essential oils 'neat' or undiluted (such as lavender and chamomile), it is always ideal to use a carrier oil with your essential oils to avoid having an adverse effect or skin irritation.

Carrier oils provide the much-needed lubrication, allowing hands to move freely over the skin, helping with the absorption of essential oils into the body. Choose a carrier oil that is light, non-sticky and that can effectively penetrate the skin. Always check the label to make sure it's 100% pure, unrefined and cold-pressed.

CARRIER OILS DIRECTORY

With the vast selection of carrier oils, each with various therapeutic benefits, choosing one will depend on the area it's being applied to, the treatment plan, and any skin sensitivities. When using oil for massage, the viscosity is an important consideration. Some carrier oils may work better than others in certain applications. For example, grapeseed oil is generally very thin while olive oil is much thicker, and others such as sunflower and sweet almond have viscosities halfway between these extremes. You can easily blend carrier oils to combine their properties of viscosity, absorption rate, and benefits. Don't forget to take into consideration the color of your carrier oil when creating a particular recipe where it may affect the outcome of the product; otherwise, for general blending purposes the color of your carrier oil won't matter.

TIP: When shopping for a good quality carrier oil, make sure it's cold-pressed so that all of its natural qualities have been retained.

Almond Oil is one of the most useful, practical and moderately priced carrier oils available. It is ideal for all skin types as it moisturizes and reconditions the skin with its satiny smooth texture. This pale-yellow oil quickly absorbs into the skin, leaving your skin feeling soft and non-greasy. Sweet almond provides relief from itching, soreness, dryness, inflammation, and is especially beneficial for eczema. As a lightly nutty refined oil rich in fatty acids, proteins and vitamin D, it is everyone's favorite massage base oil for loosening stiff muscles and achy joints.

Dilution: Can be used at 100%.

Apricot Kernel Oil is pale yellow in color and has a light texture, is easily absorbed and moisturizes both the body and face thoroughly. Extracted from the kernel of apricot fruit, it contains vitamin E, which is particularly suitable for mature skin. Vitamins A and B help in healing and rejuvenating skin cells. It is ideal for all skin types, especially for sensitive, inflamed and dry skin. Apricot seeds are well known for the presence of amygdalin, as well as vitamin B-17 and laetrile, which is a compound considered to have the potential to kill cancer cells without causing any damage to surrounding healthy cells, and lower blood pressure. Studies reveal that the consumption of apricot seeds helped in the lowering of both systolic and diastolic blood pressure in people with high blood pressure.

Dilution: Can be used at 100% or as a blend with other carrier oils such as sweet almond oil for a massage at 10% dilution.

Argan Oil comes from Morocco with over 80% unsaturated fatty acids and essential fats. It contains high amounts of vitamin E and is extremely resistant to oxidation. This cold-pressed oil is considered a treat for mature skin and valued for its nutritive, cosmetic and medicinal properties. Researchers have concluded daily consumption of argan oil can help prevent various cancers, cardiovascular disease, and obesity. Its medicinal uses also include rheumatism and healing burns. Argan oil is sometimes mixed with pomegranate seed oil due to its anti-oxidizing properties.

Dilution: Can be used at 100% or diluted with other carrier oils such as rosehip seed, coconut or apricot kernel as a blend.

Avocado Oil is rich in lecithin, vitamins, A, B1, B2, D, and E. It also contains amino acids, sterols, and pantothenic acid. It is known to delay aging as it is rich in essential fatty acids. Avocado quickly penetrates the skin, acts as a sunscreen and helps in cell regeneration. For skin that has been exposed to the sun, mix zinc oxide in half a bottle of avocado oil and apply. Avocado is greatly praised for those who suffer from skin problems such as eczema, psoriasis, and other skin disorders. The antioxidants and beta-sitosterol found in avocados help to reduce the risk of heart disease and cancer while maintaining eye health in aging adults. Avocados are also rich in monounsaturated fats, which help balance cholesterol levels. An essential nutrient for bone and cardiovascular health, the magnesium found in an avocado is also known to reduce migraines and prevent type II diabetes. The Omega-3 fatty acids in avocados may reduce inflammation, high cholesterol, high blood pressure, depression, and arthritis.

Dilution: Can be used at 100%, although in most cases, it is best mixed with another carrier oil such as sweet almond or grapeseed oil to make up 10-30% of the carrier blend.

Borage Seed Oil is naturally one of the greatest sources of GLA or gamma-linolenic acid. It improves the skin texture when used topically. Borage seed is excellent for use with children with atopic dermatitis. During the Middle Ages, borage was a traditional anti-inflammatory agent used to treat rheumatism and heart disease.

Dilution: Can be utilized at 100% as your carrier oil base, although it is recommended to use with other carrier oils up to 25% for therapeutic applications.

Carrot Seed Oil is rich in beta-carotene, and vitamins A, B, C, D, and E. This oil is known to heal dry, chapped skin, balance the moisture in the skin and condition the hair, as well. It is suitable for all skin types, especially for dry, mature skin, and is useful for face and neck treatments in reducing wrinkles. Many users find it helpful for burns, wounds, cuts, and scars. Carrot seed oil contains up to 13 percent alpha-pinene and up to 18 percent carotol. Other contents include daucol, limonene, beta-bisabolene, eugenol, vanillin, various terpenoids, coumarin, and palmitic and butyric acids. The website Drugs.com credits carrot seed oil with smooth-muscle relaxant action, as well as the ability to protect the liver, dilate blood vessels and lower blood pressure in animal studies. Carrot seed absorbs quickly into the skin and is excellent for eczema, psoriasis, and itchy scalp.

Dilution: Can be used at 100% or blended with another carrier oil at 10-25%.

Cocoa Butter is a rich and creamy butter (not a carrier oil) that must be warmed to make it liquid. It is an excellent addition to skin care products due to its high level of polyphenols, vitamins, and nutrients. It smooths, hydrates, and balances skin while providing collagen to support mature skin. Its warm aroma of cocoa is a delightful addition to lotions and creams. Cocoa butter is widely used as a treatment for pregnancy stretch marks. With its A, B1, B2, B3, C, and E vitamins, it is an excellent moisturizer for skin health. Scientists have linked cocoa butter to a reduction of blood pressure and heart disease. According to the American Heart Association, a 2006 study called "Circulation: Heart Failure" reported that middle-aged and elderly women who regularly ate a small amount of chocolate had a 32 percent lower risk of heart failure. Although scientists are not sure why, it may be due to its oleic acid or its cocoa mass polyphenol (CMP), which may protect against heart disease.

Dilution: Its firm texture makes it difficult to work in and needs to be blended with other oils to be workable. Use at a 10% dilution.

Coconut Oil (Fractionated) seems to be quickly becoming the carrier oil of choice because of its broad use in alternative medicine and healing. While it is fractionated, no change has been made chemically. Instead, its molecular structure 'fraction' has been separated, allowing it to remain liquid at room temperature, making it much more useful in aromatherapy. Coconut oil is perfect as a moisturizer for the body and conditions brittle, dry or dull hair. Because of its many health benefits, coconut oil, when used correctly, can prove beneficial in a regimen designed to lower blood pressure. Its light, easily absorbable texture gives skin a smooth satin effect with virtually no scent of its own and indefinite shelf life. Coconut oil is 92% saturated fat and contains Omega-3 fatty acids and is believed to be better for lowering blood pressure than other vegetable oils. Omega-3 fatty acids are known to widen your blood vessels and relieve inflammation of the arteries.

Dilution: Can be used at 100%.

Coconut Oil (Virgin) has an incredible balance of natural saturated fatty acids with antibacterial and antiviral properties not found in other oils. With regular use, it can improve the joint health of arthritis sufferers. Coconut oil is perfect as a skin conditioner for nearly all skin conditions and is believed to stimulate hair growth. It has a light, aromatic coconut scent that becomes solid at room temperature. For this reason, it is recommended to blend with other carrier oils in your body care products. It is fully digestible and is considered a healthy cooking oil. Several virgin coconut oils are high in antioxidants which are positively associated with reducing oxidative stress, and thus lowering blood pressure.

Dilution: Can be used alone directly but is recommended to use 10-25% dilution with other carrier oils.

Evening Primrose Oil makes a delightful addition to your carrier oil blends for arthritis. It is the perfect, lightly refined oil that can be used to moisturize, soften and soothe away dry and irritated skin and help with premature aging. Evening primrose contains gamma-linolenic acid, Omega-3 essential fats as well as other fatty acids that help the body produce Prostaglandin E1, which reduces inflammation and improves digestion. Because evening primrose oil contains Omega-6 essential fatty acids that are necessary for good health, it has been known to lower blood pressure. This oil can be taken internally. Please note this oil can go rancid quickly.

Dilution: Due to its cost, it is usually blended with other carrier oils at 10% dilution.

Flaxseed Oil is an emollient, high in essential fatty acids, vitamin E, B, and minerals. It contains the alpha-linoleic acids (ALAs), which may contribute to lowering blood pressure. Flaxseed oil eases symptoms of rheumatoid arthritis and lupus. It lubricates joints and relieves stiffness and joint pain. It is also known for its anti-inflammatory properties and for preventing scarring and stretch marks. Flaxseed oil contains both Omega-3 and Omega-6 fatty acids, which are needed for health and act as anti-inflammatories. Flaxseed oil contains the essential fatty acid alpha-linolenic acid (ALA), which the body converts into eicosapentaenoic acid (EPA) and docosahexaenoic acid (DHA), the Omega-3 fatty acids found in fish oil according to the University of Maryland Medical Center's website. ALA may reduce heart disease risks through a variety of ways, including making platelets less "sticky," reducing inflammation, promoting blood vessel health, and lessen the chance of arrhythmia (irregular heartbeat). Several human studies also suggest that diets rich in Omega-3 fatty acids (including ALA) may lower blood pressure. This golden oil will leave a greasy feeling on the skin, so it is recommended to add to other carrier oils for use in skin care products.

Dilution: Due to its heavy scent and texture, use at 10% dilution with another carrier oil or carrier oil blend.

Grapeseed Oil is a pleasing, light green and odorless oil, useful as a base oil for many creams, lotions and as a carrier oil. Grapeseed oil is pressed from the seeds of a grape and contains OPCs, flavonoids, vitamin E, resveratrol, and fatty acids. It is non-allergenic and has very high levels of linoleic acid, with traces of proanthocyanidins, which are very potent antioxidants. It is reportedly helpful in reducing stretch marks. It is used as an alternative treatment for conditions such as diabetes, hemorrhoids, cancers, high cholesterol, edema, and high blood pressure. A study conducted at the University of California at Davis found that grapeseed extract helped control blood pressure. It is especially beneficial for all skin types because of its natural non-allergenic properties. Grapeseed works well, especially when other oils do not absorb well, without leaving a greasy feeling after application. Slightly astringent, it tightens and tones the skin and alleviates acne. Grapeseed makes an ideal carrier oil for body massage bases. Saturation takes longer than some other carrier oils.

Dilution: Can be used at 100%.

Hemp Seed Oil is a hidden treasure of fatty acids, including ALA and GLA, that makes it possibly one of the most nourishing oils available. An analysis shows it contains linoleic acid, alpha and gamma linolenic acid (Omega-6), palmitic acid, stearic acid, and oleic acid. These essential fatty acids help ward off various age-related diseases and osteoarthritis. Hemp oil has been scientifically proven to improve dermatitis symptoms, reduce blood clots and high blood pressure. Like evening primrose, it is supportive of reducing inflammation, which makes it useful for arthritis and autoimmune disorders. It also stimulates hair and nail growth and makes a superb skin moisturizer. Hemp oil contains many healing and regenerative properties and may be applied topically to restore vital organs, as well as skin conditions. Research shows it is beneficial in reducing blood clots and high blood pressure. This rich, slightly green, nutty-flavored oil can be taken internally but should be refrigerated.

Dilution: Can be used at 100% or blended with other carrier oils at 20% dilution for massage purposes.

Jojoba Oil is bright and golden in color and is known as one of the best oils (actually a liquid wax) for hair and skin. It penetrates the skin quickly and is excellent for skin nourishment and for healing inflamed skin, psoriasis, eczema, or any dermatitis. Jojoba controls acne and oily skin and makes a terrific scalp cleanser as excess sebum dissolves in jojoba. It is suitable for all skin types and promotes a healthy, glowing complexion by gently unclogging the pores and lifting embedded impurities. It makes a good base oil for treating rheumatism and arthritis because of its anti-inflammatory actions. Jojoba is suitable for all aromatherapy uses other than a full-body massage. And, because of the oil's antioxidants, it does not become rancid and can even prevent rancidity in other oils.

Dilution: Can be used at 100% but due to its price, many use a 10% dilution with other carrier oils.

Olive Oil (Extra Virgin) is light to medium green in color, with a slightly dense texture. It is very soothing and carries disinfecting and healing properties. Olive oil is quite legendary since it has been used over the centuries for multiple purposes, but due to its overpowering scent, this oil does not work well for massages. However, it is beneficial in some lotions for burns or scars. Olive is very helpful for dry, damaged or split hair and is soothing for inflamed skin such as eczema. It has been proven to be very beneficial for rheumatic conditions and protects the body against harmful free-radical cell damage. Traditionally, olive oil has been used for stomach disorders, stimulates bile production, promotes pancreatic secretions and may even protect against stomach ulcers. Olive oil is reported to improve inflammatory markers and reduce oxidative stress in individuals with rheumatoid arthritis. The antihypertensive effects of olive oil are so powerful many users eliminated their need for blood pressure-lowering medications in just six months, according to a recent study. The "virgin" indicates it comes from the first pressing of the fruit. The "extra" means it comes from a single source. Extra virgin olive oil is particularly useful for high blood pressure because it contains more vitamin E than virgin, pure or extra light varieties.

Dilution: Can be used at 100% or 25-50% dilution with another carrier oil blend.

Safflower Oil has a slightly nutty aroma and is rich in an Omega-6 group of essential fatty acids, oleic acid, palmitic acid, linoleic acid, and linolenic acid as well as Vitamin E. It has the highest percentage of unsaturated fats of all vegetable oils. Because of its light texture, safflower oil is suitable for body massage. It has diuretic properties and is helpful for painful arthritis, inflamed joints, bruises, and sprains. This oil is also great for skin allergies and is beneficial for people who suffer from arteriosclerosis and is an excellent choice for those who want to improve the health of their cardiovascular system. This oil oxidizes quickly. Safflower can be used in massage blends.

Dilution: Can be used at 100% or diluted with another carrier oil blend.

Sesame Oil has a rich golden color with a bold, nutty flavor. It is a warm oil that is used for conditions such as eczema, psoriasis, and arthritis. Sesame oil is active with Vitamin A and E, minerals and lecithin. Research has shown sesame oil enriches the blood, stimulates the blood platelet count, and is effective against spleen disorders. One website reported, "It is almost as effective as a drug for bringing down high blood pressure, and the oils also improve cholesterol levels." It is high in calcium and makes an ideal laxative for those who suffer from digestive disorders. It works great as an all-over body moisturizer or massage oil. Because of its relatively stable shelf life, it is excellent in body care products and facial blends. However, it needs to be mixed with another carrier oil that inhibits oxidation or an essential oil such as benzoin. Sesame spreads easily all over the skin and leaves no greasy feeling.

Dilution: Use at 10% dilution with another carrier oil or carrier oil blend.

Shea Butter is a thick, lustrous butter (not a carrier oil) with great therapeutic properties. It contains powerful anti-inflammatory properties that can reduce swelling and pain. Research found that people who used shea in a study experienced significant decreases in markers for inflammation and cartilage degradation compared to the control group. It leaves the skin feeling smooth and healthy and combats many skin conditions including dermatitis, eczema, burns, dry skin and more. Shea butter has a very cream-like consistency so you may want to warm and blend with other carrier oils for a thinner or liquid consistency if desired.

Dilution: Can be used at 100% or diluted at 25-25% with another carrier oil for blending purposes.

Walnut Oil makes an excellent emollient with moisturizing properties for dry, aged, and irritated skin. This pale-yellow oil works as a balancing agent for the nervous system. A study published in the Journal of the American College of Nutrition examined walnuts and walnut oils, which contain polyunsaturated fats and their influence on blood pressure at rest and under stress and found it helps the body cope with stress by lowering resting blood pressure and blood pressure responses to stress. Previous studies showed that Omega-3 fatty acids—like the alpha-linolenic acid found in walnuts and flax seeds—can reduce low-density lipoproteins (LDL) and may reduce c-reactive protein and other markers of inflammation. Walnut oil can be used for massage and aromatherapy. However, it should be diluted with another carrier oil.

Dilution: Use at 10-25% dilution with another carrier oil or carrier oil blend.

DO NOT USE THESE

Mineral oil and petroleum jelly should never be used as a carrier oil in therapeutic blending. These are derivatives of petroleum production from gasoline and are not of natural botanical origins. Many commercially-based cosmetics and moisturizers contain mineral oil such as baby oil because it is inexpensive to manufacture. It prevents toxins from escaping the body through perspiration and is believed to also prevent the body from adequately absorbing vitamins and utilizing them, including essential oil absorption.

DILUTION RATE FOR YOUR ARTHRITIS BLENDS

When creating an essential oil blend for arthritis, you will need to take into consideration the percentage of dilution with a carrier oil. Be careful to dilute correctly to make sure your blend is safe to use and doesn't waste your precious essential oil.

The following dilution rate chart shows you the percentage of pure therapeutic essential oil to use with the number of drops of carrier oil (vegetable oil) and will help you convert essential and carrier oil measurements. Use a measuring cup or spoon for carrier oils and pipettes for measuring your essential oils.

It is important to dilute your essential oil blend with a suitable carrier oil so that you can use it on the skin over a part of the body. There are several different carrier oils as mentioned earlier, such as Sweet Almond, cold-pressed Extra Virgin Olive, Grapeseed Extract, Jojoba, etc. You will want to select the best one for your condition and skin type. Carrier oils can be purchased at a natural health food store or grocery but check labels to make sure the one you select is cold-pressed and is suitable for use on the skin.

In general, most essential oils should be diluted between 1%-5% with a carrier oil. For topical formulas, you will typically use 1-3% concentration of essential oils (in some cases up to 5-10%). This is 6-24 drops of essential oil per ounce of carrier. Therapeutic massage blends will contain between 1%-5% essential oils. However, each essential oil will have a different number of drops per milliliter, so to be more exact in your measuring, you will want to consider this, too.

For instance, if you use two to three drops of pure essential oil, you will dilute by adding about a teaspoon of carrier oil. This should be cut in half for children and senior citizens.

SIMPLE EVERYDAY DILUTION CHART

2-3 drops of Essential Oil per teaspoon of Carrier Oil

7-8 drops of Essential Oil per Tablespoon of Carrier Oil

15 drops of Essential Oil per ounce (30ml) of Carrier Oil

1 drop of essential oil = 1 tsp. of carrier oil for 1% dilution

2 drops of essential oil = 1 tsp. of carrier oil for 2% dilution

3 drops of essential oil = 1 tsp. of carrier oil for 3% dilution

4 drops of essential oil = 1 tsp. of carrier oil for 4% dilution

5 drops of essential oil = 1 tsp. of carrier oil for 5% dilution

Essential Oil	To	Carrier Oil
1 drop		¼ teaspoon
2-5 drops		1 teaspoon
4-10 drops		2 teaspoons
6-15 drops		1 tablespoon
8-20 drops		4 teaspoons
12-30 drops		2 tablespoons

For general purposes, a blend is applied 6 times a day for acute conditions and 3-6 times a day for chronic complaints, or as needed.

MASSAGE OIL

When you use essential oils for a massage, you will definitely need to dilute with a carrier oil. Generally, two drops of therapeutic grade essential oil should be used per teaspoon of carrier oil (follow individual recipes when available). A full body massage takes about one to two ounces of carrier oil. Any natural carrier oil (except mineral oil) is okay to use when preparing a massage blend. As a general rule, add 10-12 drops of essential oil to 30ml of carrier oil. For children and elderly, use only 5-6 drops of essential oil to 30ml of carrier oil.

QUICK CONVERSIONS FOR DILUTION

Teaspoons to Drops

1 teaspoon = 100 drops = 1/6 ounce = 5 ml

ML Conversion to Ounces (approximate drops)

1 ml = 20-24 drops

3 ml = .10 ounces (approximately 60-72 drops)

6 ml = .20 ounces (approximately 120-144 drops)

9 ml = .30 ounces (approximately 180-216 drops)

12 ml = .40 ounces (approximately 240-288 drops)

24 ml = .80 ounces (approximately 480-576 drops)

QUICK CONVERSIONS

3 teaspoons (tsp.) = 1 tablespoon (tbsp.)

2 Tablespoons (Tbsp.) = 1 ounce (oz.)

6 teaspoons (tsp.) = 1 ounce (oz.)

10 milliliter (ml) = 1/3 ounce (oz.)

15 milliliter (ml) = 1/2 ounce (oz.)

30 milliliter (ml) = 1 ounce (oz.)

10 milliliter (ml) = approximately 300 drops

1% DILUTION RATE (APPROXIMATE)

- 1 ounce carrier oil (2 tablespoons) + 6 drops essential oil
- 2 ounces carrier oil (1/4 cup) + 12 drops essential oil
- 3 ounces carrier oil (1/3 cup) + 18 drops essential oil
- 4 ounces carrier oil (1/2 cup) + 24 drops (or 1 ml) essential oil
- 8 ounces carrier oil (1 cup) + 48 drops (or 2 ml) essential oil

2% DILUTION RATE (APPROXIMATE)

- 1 ounce carrier oil (2 tablespoons) + 12 drops essential oil
- 1 ounce carrier oil (1/4 cup) + 24 drops (or 1 ml) essential oil
- 1 ounce carrier oil (1/3 cup) + 36 drops (or 1½ ml) essential oil
- 4 ounces carrier oil (1/2 cup) + 48 drops (or 2 ml) essential oil
- 8 ounces carrier oil (1 cup) + 96 drops (or 4 ml) essential oil

3% DILUTION RATE (APPROXIMATE)

- 1 ounce carrier oil (2 tablespoons) + 18 drops essential oil
- 1 ounce carrier oil (1/4 cup) + 36 drops (or 1½ ml) essential oil
- 3 ounces carrier oil (1/3 cup) + 44 drops (or 2 ml) essential oil
- 4 ounces carrier oil (1/2 cup) + 72 drops (or 3 ml) essential oil
- 8 ounces carrier oil (1 cup) + 144 drops (or 6 ml) essential oil

5% DILUTION RATE (APPROXIMATE)

- 1 ounce carrier oil (2 tablespoons) + 1.5 ml essential oil
- 2 ounces carrier oil (1/4 cup) + 3 ml essential oil
- 3 ounces carrier oil (1/3 cup) + 4.5 ml essential oil
- 4 ounces carrier oil (1/2 cup) + 6 ml essential oil
- 8 ounces carrier oil (1 cup) + 9 ml essential oil

10% DILUTION RATE (APPROXIMATE)

- 1 ounce carrier oil (2 tablespoons) + 3 ml essential oil
- 2 ounces carrier oil (1/4 cup) + 6 ml essential oil
- 3 ounces carrier oil (1/3 cup) + 9 ml essential oil
- 4 ounces carrier oil (1/2 cup) + 12 ml essential oil
- 8 ounces carrier oil (1 cup) + 24 ml essential oil

EQUIPMENT USED FOR CREATING BLENDS FOR ARTHRITIS

Before getting started, you will want to gather the supplies you will need such as bottles, droppers, and containers. Below is a list of the necessary tools you will need to have on hand:

Glass Bottles, preferably dark, in 5ml, 10ml, and 15ml sizes with orifice reducers (plastic dropper) can be used to make topical essential oil blends.

Plastic Bottles with a pump, squirt, or screw off top are suitable for liquid soaps, shower gels, shampoos, lotions, and conditioners. You can find these in 2-ounce, 4-ounce, and 8-ounce sizes.

Plastic or Glass Spray Bottles are great to have on hand when making room sprays, facial spritzers or cleaning solutions. You will find these in 1-ounce, 2-ounce, 4-ounce, 8-ounce, and 16-ounce sizes.

Small Glass or Plastic Tubs are perfect for bath salts, facial creams, salves, scrubs or other bath blends. These come in a variety of shapes and sizes from 2-ounce to 8-ounce.

Pocket Diffusers are perfect as "personal inhalers" to carry in a pocket or purse with your favorite blend. They come with a cotton wick that saturates the essential oil inside the chamber. These are terrific for taking to work or school!

Plastic Transfer Pipettes come in different sizes and lengths for easy and precise drop measuring. They are ideal for filling small vials and for measure dropping small amounts of oils. Use these when you want to transfer oil from a large bottle into smaller bottles. They are for one-time use and should be thrown away to avoid cross-contamination.

Clear Mini Atomizers are perfect for trips. You can use these to make and share with friends and family (1ml or 2ml sizes work best).

You will need waterproof labels for your bottles, and you will want them in all shapes and sizes. Visit Online Labels for a wide variety of sizes at http://www.onlinelabels.com/.

Items such as bottles and pipettes are available online at SKS Bottle & Packaging and Rachel's Supply.

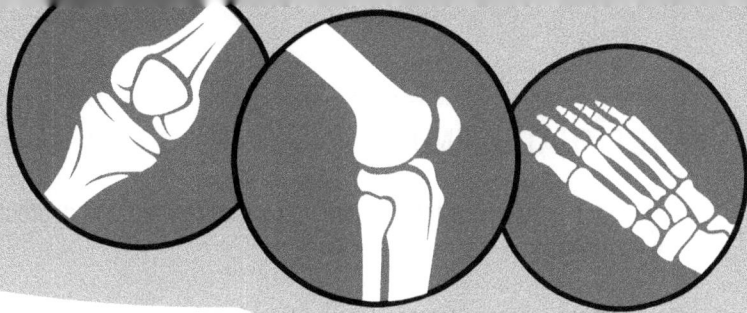

RECIPES

In this chapter, you will find an assortment of recipes to choose from in treating symptoms of arthritis. Since there are so many types of arthritis, you will want to try different combinations of oils for improved efficacy. Results will vary from person to person. You may also want to come up with your own blend based on the oils you have on hand.

TOP THAT BLEND

This fast-acting blend will significantly reduce pain and depression associated with arthritis.

WHAT YOU WILL NEED:
4 drops Lavender essential oil
2 drops Marjoram essential oil
4 drops Eucalyptus essential oil
2 drops Rosemary essential oil
2 drops Peppermint essential oil
40 drops Jojoba oil
½ ounce Apricot oil
½ ounce Almond oil
2-ounce glass bottle
Funnel
Pipette

WHAT TO DO:
1. In a glass bottle, add essential oils using a pipette.
2. Using a funnel, add carrier oils.
3. Replace cap and shake to blend.
4. Use as needed on affected areas.

MASSAGE JOINT PAIN RELIEF

For instant relief, try making this potent massage oil for joint pain.

WHAT YOU WILL NEED:
3 drops Peppermint essential oil
5 drops Clove essential oil
5 drops Frankincense essential oil
5 drops Rose essential oil
½ cup Sesame oil
4-ounce dark glass bottle
Funnel
Pipette

WHAT TO DO:
1. In a small glass bowl, add your essential oils and stir to blend.
2. Remove cap from the glass bottle, then pour your carrier oil (sesame) into the bottle using a funnel.
3. Next, add the essential oils to the bottle using a pipette.
4. Replace cap and shake to blend.
5. To use, pour ½ teaspoon out into your palm and gently rub into and/or around joints. Massage the area for five minutes. Repeat twice a day.
6. Store in a cool, dark place.

WD-40 BLEND

This essential oil blend helps with the pain associated with arthritis and the depression that goes with it. It is based on a study conducted on forty hospital patients in South Korea that found these oils "significantly decreased both the pain score and the depression score of the experimental group compared with the control group."

WHAT YOU WILL NEED:

4 drops Myrrh essential oil

2 drops Marjoram essential oil

4 drops Eucalyptus essential oil

2 drops Turmeric essential oil

2 drops Wintergreen essential oil

1 tablespoon Almond oil

1 tablespoon Apricot oil

1 teaspoon Jojoba oil

2-ounce Glass bottle

Funnel

Pipette

WHAT TO DO:

1. In a glass bottle, use a funnel to add carrier oils (almond, apricot, jojoba).

2. Add essential oils and replace the cap. Shake to blend well.

3. Apply blend to affected joints as needed throughout the day.

ORANGE-GINGER THAI MASSAGE BLEND

This massage blend is based on a placebo-controlled and double-blind study conducted at a senior citizen center in Hong Kong. The results were astounding. Pain and stiffness gone!

WHAT YOU WILL NEED:

5 drops Orange essential oil

5 drops Ginger essential oil

1 tablespoon Olive oil

15ml glass bottle

Pipette

Funnel

WHAT TO DO:

1. Add carrier oil (olive oil) to the glass bottle.
2. Add essential oils. Replace cap and shake to mix well.
3. To use, rub oil blend on affected areas and joints to alleviate pain. To use as a massage oil, ask a friend or family member to perform an aromatic massage on you.

ARTHRO TUNE-UP (RHEUMATOID)

This essential oil blend will increase circulation and help alleviate arthritis and rheumatic conditions.

WHAT YOU WILL NEED:
2 drops Wintergreen essential oil

2 drops Marjoram essential oil

2 drops Peppermint essential oil

2 drops Lavender essential oil

2 drops Oregano essential oil

2 drops Cypress essential oil

2 drops Helichrysum essential oil

1 ounce Carrier oil

WHAT TO DO:
1. Add carrier oil into the 1-ounce bottle.
2. Add essential oils. Replace cap and shake to mix well.
3. To use, rub ½ to 1 teaspoon oil blend to the affected area as needed. To use as a massage oil, ask a friend or family member to perform an aromatic massage on you.

RHEUMATOID ARTHRITIS FOOT ROLL-ON BLEND

Oregano and clove bud essential oils are strong essential oils, so its recommended to use on the soles of the feet.

WHAT YOU WILL NEED:

3 drops Oregano essential oil

3 drops Clove bud essential oil

1 tablespoon Carrier oil

15ml glass roll-on bottle

WHAT TO DO:

1. Add carrier to 15ml glass roll-on bottle. Be sure to leave a little space at the top for essential oils.
2. Add drops of essential oils to bottle. Pop roller ball into place and replace the cap. Shake to mix well.
3. To use, use roll-on on the bottom of the feet twice daily.

ESSENTIALLY AWESOME ARTHRITIS MASSAGE BLEND

Massage this blend into affected areas so that it penetrates deeply.

WHAT YOU WILL NEED:

3 drops Black Pepper essential oil

3 drops Roman Chamomile essential oil

3 drops Lavender essential oil

3 drops Lemon essential oil

3 drops Rosemary essential oil

1 ounce Jojoba carrier oil or unscented cream

WHAT TO DO:

1. Add jojoba carrier oil to a 1-ounce bottle.
2. Add essential oils. Replace cap and shake to mix well.
3. To use, massage into your affected areas or use in the bath.

MAX PAIN RELIEF FORMULA

This ultra-strength topical blend eases muscular, joint and back pain.

WHAT YOU WILL NEED:
6 drops Helichrysum italicum essential oil
4 drops Marjoram essential oil
2 drops Juniper Berry essential oil
4 drops Birch Bark or Wintergreen essential oil
3 drops German Chamomile essential oil
3 drops Lavender essential oil
3 drops Ginger Root essential oil
2 ounces Carrier oil of choice
2-ounce bottle

WHAT TO DO:
1. Add carrier oil to the 2-ounce bottle.
2. Add essential oils. Replace cap and shake to mix well.
3. To use, add 1 tablespoon to 1 cup sea salts to use in the bath.

ANTI-ARTHRITIS PAIN RELIEF BATH OIL

Warning: this blend is deeply relaxing. Add mixture to a warm, running bath and soak in it before bed.

WHAT YOU WILL NEED:

15 drops Lavender essential oil

8 drops Clary Sage essential oil

7 drops Ylang Ylang essential oil

2 ounce Sweet Almond carrier oil

2-ounce bottle

WHAT TO DO:

1. Add sweet almond carrier to a 2-ounce bottle.
2. Add essential oils. Replace cap and shake well to mix.
3. To use, add 1-2 tablespoons into bath water and soak for 15 minutes. Or add oil with Epsom or sea salts and soak for 15 minutes.

HEALING HOT PEPPER LINIMENT

Some like it hot, and this one is!

WHAT YOU WILL NEED:
1 cup fresh Ginger; finely chopped, sliced or grated
1 teaspoon Cayenne pepper
1 teaspoon Vegetable Glycerin
2 1/2 cups unflavored Vodka
1-quart glass jar
Plastic wrap
Coffee filter
Strainer

WHAT TO DO:
1. Place ginger, glycerin, and cayenne pepper into a glass jar and add vodka.
2. Place plastic wrap over the top of the jar to prevent the metal jar top from touching the contents of the jar.
3. Shake jar for 30 seconds to blend contents.
4. Store jar for 4 weeks in a cool and dark place. Shake every day for 15-20 seconds.
5. After 4 weeks, strain all contents through a coffee filter in a strainer.
6. To use, apply a small amount of ointment to affected areas.

ARTHRITIS BATH BLEND

Soak in infused sea salts for soothing relief.

WHAT YOU WILL NEED:
3 drops Fennel essential oil

2 drops Cypress essential oil

1 ounce Jojoba oil

1-ounce bottle

WHAT TO DO:
1.   Add jojoba to bottle.
2.   Add essential oils. Replace cap and shake well to mix.
3.   To use, add sea salts and several drops of the bath blend to the bath. Use daily for two weeks.

REGENERATIVE ARTHRITIS MASSAGE OIL

Scientific research supports that both of these oils contain regenerative properties.

WHAT YOU WILL NEED:

10 drops Eucalyptus essential oil

10 drops Helichrysum italicum essential oil

1 teaspoon Sesame oil

15ml glass roll-on bottle

WHAT TO DO:

1. Add sesame oil to glass roll-on bottle.

2. Add essential oils. Replace cap and shake well to mix.

3. Apply to affected areas once a day.

JUNIOR'S ARTHRITIS BLEND

This recipe works for anyone but contains a few extra ingredients for children who suffer from arthritis.

WHAT YOU WILL NEED:

5 drops Ginger Root essential oil

5 drops Marjoram essential oil

5 drops Myrtle essential oil

2 drops Clove Bud essential oil

4 drops Helichrysum italicum essential oil

2 ounces Sesame oil

2-ounce bottle

WHAT TO DO:

1. Add sesame oil to the 2-ounce bottle.
2. Add essential oils. Replace cap and shake well to mix.
3. Apply ½ teaspoon to affected areas.

INFLAMED JOINTS BATH BLEND

There is nothing better than a warm bath with soothing oils such as Roman and German chamomile, lavender, and eucalyptus.

WHAT YOU WILL NEED:

10 drops German Chamomile essential oil

5 drops Roman Chamomile essential oil

10 drops Lavender essential oil

10 drops Eucalyptus citriodora essential oil

2 ounces Almond oil

2-ounce bottle

WHAT TO DO:

1. Add almond oil to the bottle.

2. Add essential oils. Replace cap and shake well to mix.

3. Massage a small amount of oil on the inflamed area and then take a bath.

MASSAGE OIL FOR SCIATICA

If you have radiating pains down the back of your leg, or pain in your lower back or buttocks making it uncomfortable to sit, walk or sleep, this blend is for you. It combines many active ingredients that relieve burning pains and tingling sensations.

WHAT YOU WILL NEED:

1 ounce St. John's Wort oil

1 ounce Extra Virgin Olive oil

5 drops Geranium essential oil

3 drops Peppermint essential oil

10 drops Lavender essential oil

2-ounce bottle

WHAT TO DO:

1. Add St. John's Wort oil and olive oil to the 2-ounce bottle.
2. Add essential oils. Replace cap and shake to mix well.
3. Let sit 24 hours before use. Apply to affected areas after a bath or shower.

ICY-HOT ANALGESIC MASSAGE RUB

Get immediate pain relief with these powerful analgesic oils.

WHAT YOU WILL NEED:
10 drops Eucalyptus essential oil

10 drops Peppermint essential oil

7 drops Cajeput essential oil (possible substitutes: Ginger, Tea Tree, or Rosemary)

2 drops Cinnamon Bark essential oil

2 drops Clove Bud essential oil

2 ounces Jojoba oil

2-ounce bottle

WHAT TO DO:
1. Add jojoba to a 2-ounce bottle.
2. Add essential oils. Replace cap and shake to mix well.
3. Let sit for 24 hours. To use, apply to affected areas in small doses.

TENSION BLEND

This blend will help resolve tension, soreness, and stiffness.

WHAT YOU WILL NEED:
2 ounce Extra Virgin Olive oil
10 drops Black Pepper essential oil
12 drops Coriander essential oil
6 drops White Grapefruit essential oil
2 drops Ginger Root essential oil
2-ounce bottle

WHAT TO DO:
1. Add olive oil to the bottle.
2. Add essential oils. Replace cap and shake well to mix.
3. Let sit for 24 hours. Apply to affected areas after bath or shower.

ST. JOHN'S WORT BLEND

This traditional recipe has been used for centuries for arthritic relief.

WHAT YOU WILL NEED:
3 cups freshly wilted St. John's Wort flowering tops
3-4 cups Extra Virgin Olive oil
2,000 IU Vitamin E oil
4-6 drops Essential oil of your choice
1-quart jar
Plastic wrap
Coffee filter
Strainer

WHAT TO DO:
1. Put herbs into a quart jar and fill the jar with olive oil leaving 1 inch of space.
2. Stir to remove any bubbles and make sure all herbs are submerged.
3. Place plastic wrap over the top of the jar to make sure the metal lid is not touching contents.
4. Place jar in a warm place. Shake 30 seconds a day for 4 weeks.
5. Strain everything through a coffee filter and a strainer.
6. Discard all herbs.
7. Store in a dark glass jar.
8. Use by massaging into the affected area. Allow to soak in before 5-10 minutes.

WARMING PAIN RELIEF BLEND

Adding warmth to your joints eases the pain, allowing healing to take place.

WHAT YOU WILL NEED:
4 drops Bay Leaf essential oil
6 drops Helichrysum essential oil
4 drops Clove Bud essential oil
6 drops Roman Chamomile essential oil
6 drops Ginger Root essential oil
6 drops Rosemary essential oil
6 drops Lavender essential oil
2 tablespoons Jojoba oil
2 teaspoons Castor oil
2 teaspoons St. John's Wort oil
1 teaspoon Calendula oil
2-ounce bottle

WHAT TO DO:
1. Add jojoba, castor oil, St. John's Wort, and calendula to bottle.
2. Add essential oils. Replace cap and shake well to mix.
3. Let sit for 24 hours. Apply to affected areas in small doses.

REDUCING ARTHRITIC INFLAMMATION BLEND

Its name says it all! Reduce inflammation with essential oils like marjoram, eucalyptus, and lavender.

WHAT YOU WILL NEED:

2 drops Eucalyptus essential oil

2 drops Marjoram essential oil

1 drop Lavender essential oil

1 drop Rosemary essential oil

1 drop Peppermint essential oil

1 ounce Carrier oil of your choice (Coconut, Sesame Seed, Sweet Almond, Jojoba, Grapeseed, Macadamia)

1-ounce bottle

WHAT TO DO:

1. Add carrier of your choice to the 1-ounce bottle.

2. Add essential oils. Replace cap and shake well to mix.

3. Apply to affected areas as needed.

SOOTHING MUSCLE ROLL-ON BLEND

This sports blend will carry you away to the great outdoors.

WHAT YOU WILL NEED:
3 drops Wintergreen essential oil
3 drops Peppermint essential oil
2 drops Juniper Berry essential oil
2 drops Lemongrass essential oil
15ml Carrier oil of choice
15ml roll-on bottle

WHAT TO DO:
1. Add carrier of choice into the 15ml roll-on bottle.
2. Add essential oils. Replace cap and shake well to mix.
3. Apply to sore muscles and massage to help reduce inflammation.

CALMING INFLAMMATION RELIEF ROLL-ON BLEND

Convenience is what this blend is all about. Have on hand and use as needed.

WHAT YOU WILL NEED:
10 drops Lavender essential oil
5 drops Rosemary essential oil
5 drops Eucalyptus essential oil
5 drops Birch essential oil
3 drops Peppermint essential oil
Carrier oil of your choice
8ml roll on bottle

WHAT TO DO:
1. Add the carrier of your choice to 8ml roll-on bottle.
2. Add essential oils. Replace cap and shake well to mix.
3. Apply to affected areas as needed.

RHEUMATOID ARTHRITIS CAPSULE BLEND

This blend is for those who prefer taking oils in capsule form as a dietary supplement.

WHAT YOU WILL NEED:

4 drops Frankincense essential oil

4 drops Balsam Fir essential oil

4 drops Copaiba essential oil

1 drop Nutmeg essential oil

Empty capsules

WHAT TO DO:

1. In a small glass bowl, add each essential oil. Stir to mix well.
2. Using a pipette, add oil to the capsule.
3. Take twice daily.

TURMERIC TEA

This simple recipe has only five ingredients and is known as "liquid gold." It's no wonder since it can reduce inflammation and strengthen your bones.

WHAT YOU WILL NEED:
1 cup coconut milk
1 cup water
1 tablespoon ghee
1 tablespoon honey
1 teaspoon turmeric (powder or grated root)
Saucepan

WHAT TO DO:
1. Pour coconut milk and water into saucepan and warm for 2 minutes.
2. Add butter, raw honey, and turmeric powder. Heat for another 2 minutes.
3. Stir and pour into glasses.

JOINT RELIEF BATH BLEND

Epsom salts, baking soda, and oils are the winning combination for a deserving and relaxing bath.

WHAT YOU WILL NEED:

3 drops Cypress essential oil

4 drops Lavender essential oil

5 drops Rosemary essential oil

6 drops Wintergreen essential oil

1 cup Epsom or Dead Sea Salts

1 cup Baking Soda

WHAT TO DO:

1. Mix essential oils.
2. In another container, combine Epsom salts and baking soda. Stir well.
3. Pour oils into salts and mix well.
4. To use, add ½ cup of blend into warm water and soak for 20 minutes.

FRESH CITRUS SORE JOINT MASSAGE BLEND

This citrusy-herbal blend goes right to work. Rub on achy joints as needed.

WHAT YOU WILL NEED:
2 drops Black Pepper essential oil (optional)
3 drops Ginger essential oil
4 drops Clove Bud essential oil
3 drops Rosemary essential oil
5 drops Marjoram essential oil
3 drops Bergamot essential oil
1 ounce Carrier oil (your choice: Almond or Jojoba)
1-ounce bottle

WHAT TO DO:
1. Add carrier oil to the bottle.
2. Add essential oils. Replace cap and shake well to mix.
3. Apply to affected areas as needed.

ANTI-INFLAMED JOINT BLEND

Use this blend to reduce swelling on contact.

WHAT YOU WILL NEED:
2 drops Peppermint essential oil
2 drops Lemon essential oil
5 drops Eucalyptus essential oil
5 drops Rosemary essential oil
6 drops Lavender essential oil
1 ounce Carrier oil (Sesame or another oil)
1-ounce bottle

WHAT TO DO:
1. Add carrier to bottle.
2. Add essential oils. Replace cap and shake well to mix.
3. Massage ½ teaspoon on affected areas for a week.

EASY DOES IT BLEND

This powerful blend of essential oils knocks it out of the park with quick relief.

WHAT YOU WILL NEED:
4 drops Juniper Berry essential oil
4 drops Geranium essential oil
5 drops German Chamomile essential oil
3 drops Thyme essential oil
2 drops Frankincense essential oil
1 ounce Carrier oil (Grapeseed or another oil)
1-ounce bottle

WHAT TO DO:
1. Add carrier oil to the bottle.
2. Add essential oils. Replace cap and shake well to mix.
3. Use ½ teaspoon on affected areas.

ARTHRO RUB BLEND

This blend will bring "icy-hot" relief immediately.

WHAT YOU WILL NEED:

3 drops Wintergreen essential oil

3 drops Lemongrass essential oil

3 drops Frankincense essential oil

3 drops Eucalyptus essential oil

1 ounce Fractionated Coconut oil

1-ounce bottle

WHAT TO DO:

1. Add coconut oil into the bottle.
2. Add essential oils. Replace cap and shake well to mix.
3. To use, massage onto painful areas as needed. Apply every 30 minutes until relief is achieved.

SORE MUSCLE SALVE

Salves are great to have on hand and easy to use without the mess.

WHAT YOU WILL NEED:
10 drops Wintergreen essential oil

10 drops Lemongrass essential oil

10 drops Marjoram essential oil

10 drops Lavender essential oil

1 tablespoon Beeswax

4 tablespoons Carrier oil (Coconut, Almond, or another favorite)

Small tin or container with a lid

WHAT TO DO:
1. In a saucepan, gently melt beeswax and add carrier oil over low heat. Stir frequently.
2. Remove from heat, and allow to cool for 1 minute.
3. Stir in essential oils and mix well.
4. While mixture is still soft, pour into small storage tins or containers.
5. Allow to cool completely before replacing lid.
6. For use, apply to sore muscles for aches and pains.

SORE MUSCLE SOAK BLEND

Soaking in a hot bath brings soothing comfort. Try this one before bed and wake up more invigorated!

WHAT YOU WILL NEED:

4 drops Black Pepper essential oil

2 drops Rosemary essential oil

1 drop Ginger essential oil

½ cup Epsom salts

WHAT TO DO:

1. Combine Epsom salts and essential oils in a storage container.
2. To use, add to warm bath water and soak for 30 minutes.

WARM PAIN RELIEF BATH

Pain, which is closely related to inflammation, can be slightly moderate to severe. Try this remedy to ease pain and discomfort.

WHAT YOU WILL NEED:

4 drops Ginger essential oil

6 drops Orange essential oil

6 drops Clove essential oil

2 drops Lavender essential oil

½ cup Baking Soda

1 cup Epsom or Sea Salts

Container to store salts

WHAT TO DO:

1. In a storage container, add dry ingredients (sea salts and baking soda). Mix well.
2. Add essential oils and stir to mix into salts.
3. When ready to use, add ½ cup salts into the tub under running water. Swish water to dissolve salt blend. Soak in the tub for 20 minutes.

RHEUMATIC PAIN RELIEF ROLL-ON BLEND

Carry this with you in your purse or pocket for quick relief on the go!

WHAT YOU WILL NEED:
2 drops Spikenard essential oil

2 drops Lavender essential oil

4 drops Ginger essential oil

4 drops White Fir essential oil

1 tablespoon Fractionated Coconut oil (or another carrier oil)

8ml roll-on bottle

Funnel

WHAT TO DO:
1. Add carrier to 8ml roll-on bottle.
2. Add essential oils. Replace cap and shake well.
3. Apply to affected areas.

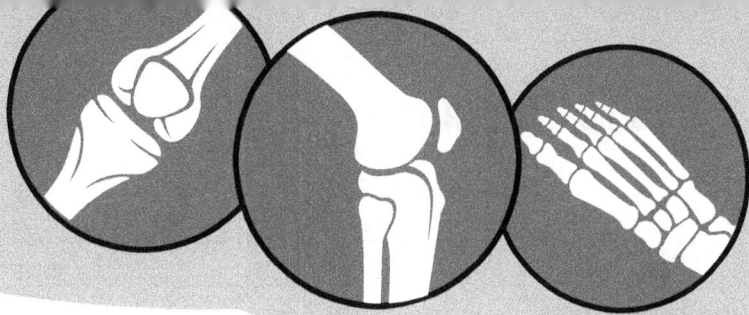

CREATING BLENDS FOR ARTHRITIS

Coming up with your own essential oil blend for reducing pain and inflammation due to arthritis is easy to do when you follow the blend by note technique. Your essential oil blend will contain one or more oils from each of these categories: Base note, Middle note, and Top note (see chart on next page). Some apothecaries recommend using a fourth note, a fixative or bridge note such as lavender, chamomile, marjoram or myrrh. The bridge is what helps the other three oils meld.

Often Vitamin E oil is used for topical blends. The following chart contains essential oils that are known to be beneficial for arthritis. Each essential oil is listed by its common name and note classification: Top, Middle, and Base.

OILS FOR ARTHRITIS

TOP	MIDDLE	BASE
Basil	Black Pepper	Benzoin
Bergamot	Roman Chamomile	Cedarwood
Camphor, White	German Chamomile	Cypress
Cilantro	Clary Sage	Frankincense
Coriander	Clove Bud	Ginger
Eucalyptus	Juniper Berry	Myrrh
Fennel (sweet)	Lavender	Rose
Galbanum	Lavandin	Sandalwood
Hyssop	Marjoram	Turmeric
Lemongrass	Rosemary	Vetiver
Lime	Spruce	
Peppermint	Wintergreen	
Scotch Pine	Yarrow	
Thyme		

Some oils made fall into more than one category. This is possible because of the many components essential oils possess and the synergy effect a blend might draw out of that oil. For this reason, you may find aromatherapists disagree to which group they fall in. However, don't let this trouble you. Instead, make this work to your advantage when creating your therapeutic blends. For instance, there may come a time when you have several middle note essential oils on hand to choose from, but no top notes for your particular condition. In this case, you could use an essential oil that may be a top note and middle note as your top note and choose a different oil as your middle note. Follow this simply as a guide when orchestrating your blends and let your nose have the final say.

Top Notes are oils that have a light, fresh aroma. It is the first scent you smell after applying a blend to the skin. Although they quickly evaporate, the top note is what gives us our first impression of a blend. Familiar top notes include lemon, bergamot, orange, lime, and other citrus oils. Most top notes are made up chemically of aldehydes and esters, which are generally found in oils from fruits, flowers, and leaves.

For Therapeutic Blending: Use 3 to 15 drops of a top note per 30 ml (or one ounce) carrier.

Middle Notes, also referred to as heart notes, are usually the inspiration for an aromatic blend and includes floral scents such as roman chamomile, lavender, or neroli. It is generally considered the heart of the blend as it often serves to cover up any unpleasant odors that may come from the base notes. Essential oils classified as middle notes are sometimes referred to as enhancers, equalizers, or balancers. Chemically, these are monoterpene alcohols found mostly in herbs and leaves. Examples of essential oil middle notes include lavender, roman chamomile, cypress, geranium, juniper berry, rosemary, and peppermint. Middle notes are what we smell when the scent from the top notes fades. This scent often evaporates after 15 seconds. The middle note can last 2-4 hours in the body and as the "heart" of the blend can play on the emotions. Middle notes are often found in flowers, leaves, and needles. They also act to bring together the top and base note as a "synergy" in a blend.

For Therapeutic Blending: Use 2 to 10 drops of a middle note per 30 ml (or one ounce) carrier.

Base Notes, usually the backbone and foundation of the blend, is what the users will remember most about a particular fragrance. The scent of base notes will last the longest in the air and are what you smell after about 30 seconds of applying it to your skin. The base note is added to the mixture first. Examples of essential oil base notes include vanilla, sandalwood, patchouli, frankincense, cinnamon, or other earthy and woodsy scents. Typically, a therapeutic blend has only one base note oil in it as it will stay the longest on the skin and can last up to 72 hours in the body. Aromatic blends can have one or more base oils to add character. Chemically speaking, base notes are made up of sesquiterpenes or diterpenes and are mainly found in roots, gums, and resins. Though therapeutic blends will typically contain one base note while aromatic blends may contain more than one, for any blend to be successful, they must have a combination of all three notes.

For Therapeutic Blending: Use 1 to 5 drops of a base note per 30 ml (or one ounce) carrier.

It is important when making an essential oil blend for your arthritis blend to mix the extracts in order starting with the base note, followed by the middle note and finally the top note. This ensures your blend will create an aroma known as a "bouquet" by staying in tune with odor intensity as well as finding notes that strike a chord and harmonize well together in therapeutic properties. Just remember, for every drop of the base note, you add 2 drops of middle note and 3 drops of the top note. This will ensure that your blend is well-rounded having all three notes, and is chemically balanced between monoterpenes, sesquiterpenes, and phenols.

TIP: Everyone is unique and what works for your condition, may not work as well for another. Be willing to try different combinations to find which oils help you the most.

MAKING YOUR FIRST ARTHRITIS BLEND

Now that you have learned about how many drops of each note to use in your essential oil blend and have checked the precautions, it's time to start blending.

1. Before you begin, gather all of the necessary equipment: bottles, pipettes, essential oils, paper towels, labels, vials, and/or containers.

2. Make sure the counter space is clean, and the area you are working in is well ventilated. You may want to put down wax paper (or a paper towel) to prevent any damage to the countertop from accidental spills. This will also make clean up much easier.

3. If you are using essential oils that are new to you, place one drop of the oil on a test strip (or small piece of paper) and wave it under your nose. Inhale the fragrance. If this fragrance is not what you had in mind, choose another oil and test again. You will want to do this with each oil until you have settled on the ones you want to use for your blend. It is a good idea to have a can of coffee grounds to smell after each fragrance to clear your palette.

4. Once you have chosen the three oils for your blend, wave all three test strips fanned out beneath your nose and see if you like it. You may not care too much, as long as it helps with pain, inflammation and other symptoms of arthritis. Keep in mind, though, if you despise the scent, you may be hesitant about using it regularly.

5. Check the safety precautions for the essential oils you have chosen to make sure there aren't any contradictions. Always take into consideration any other health conditions such as epilepsy, or any medications that may cause an adverse effect. The safety precautions must always be taken into account for

the method you choose in their usage and for the person you are formulating the blend for.

6. Choose a new, clean bottle to use. Using a pipette, extract each essential oil into the bulb to place in your bottle. You may need to squeeze more than once to get the amount you want. Remember to use a separate pipette or glass eye dropper for each of the oils used. Add your base note essential oil first, one drop at a time. This is typically the most viscous or thickest oil. Next, add the middle note essential oil, followed by the top note essential oil. Be careful to use only the exact number of drops your recipe calls for. One drop too many can alter the results. Replace the cap on the bottle and shake to mix oils.

7. Add your essential oil blend to a carrier oil (or lotion, gel, sea salts, etc.) and blend well to distribute the oils. What you use as your carrier and how much to add will depend on which method of application (Massage Blend, Bath Blend, Room Spray, etc.) you choose.

TIP: Always leave ½ inch of headspace at the top of your bottle allowing your pure essential oil blend to breathe and expand.

BASIC MASSAGE OIL BLEND RECIPE

Here is an easy-to-follow basic recipe for making a massage blend! You get to decide which essential oils to use depending on the type of massage and effect you're looking to achieve.

WHAT YOU WILL NEED:

1 ounce (30 ml) Carrier Oil, Lotion, or Gel

9-15 drops Top Note Essential Oil

6-10 drops Middle Note Essential Oil

3-5 drops Base Note Essential Oil

Plastic Bottle

WHAT TO DO:

1. Pour your carrier oil, lotion or gel into a clean bottle.
2. Add your essential oils one drop at a time, starting with your base note, followed by the middle note, and then the top note.
3. Shake well to mix oils and carrier together.
4. Add a label with name, ingredients, and date created.
5. Use two to three times a day.

BASIC BATH SALTS BLEND RECIPE

For this basic bath salts recipe, you can use Dead Sea, Himalayan, or Epsom salts. Soak in a bath with this great blend to soothe away the stress of the day. Your bath salts can be made in advance and stored in a container for convenience.

WHAT YOU WILL NEED:

2 cups Epsom Salts

1 cup Sea Salts

1 cup Baking Soda

30 drops Top Note Essential Oil

20 drops Middle Note Essential Oil

10 drops Base Note Essential Oil

Wide Mouth Jar or container

WHAT TO DO:

1. Add essential oils together in container. Stir to mix.
2. Add sea salts and mix well to saturate the salts with the oils thoroughly.
3. In a running bath, add bath salts and swish around in the tub to mix thoroughly.

TIP:

Be sure to check precautions for oils that may cause sensitivity to skin. Not recommended for children.

BASIC SALT SCRUB BLEND RECIPE

Salt scrubs are great for increasing circulation. For this basic salt scrub recipe, you can choose which salt you prefer such as Dead Sea, Himalayan, or Epsom salts. Try it for painful joints and achy muscles, too. Your salt scrub can be made fresh each time, or you may want to make some up and store in a container for when the time is right.

WHAT YOU WILL NEED:

½ cup Sea Salts

2-4 ounces Carrier Oil (your choice)

9-12 drops Top Note Essential Oil

6-8 drops Middle Note Essential Oil

3-4 drops Base Note Essential Oil

Wide Mouth Jar or container

WHAT TO DO:

1. Add carrier oil to container.
2. Add essential oils. Stir to mix well.
3. Add sea salts and mix well to saturate the salts with the oils thoroughly.
4. In the shower or bath, scrub the salt solution into the skin in upward motions toward the heart and in the direction of the lymph flow.

TIP:

Be sure to check precautions for oils that may cause sensitivity to skin. Not recommended for children.

BASIC SALVE BLEND RECIPE

Carrying a small tin in your pocket is not only convenient but is easy to use.

WHAT YOU WILL NEED:
½ - 1 cup Olive Oil or another Carrier Oil
2 teaspoons Beeswax
9 drops Top Note Essential Oil
6 drops Middle Note Essential Oil
3 drops Base Note Essential Oil
Small Jar or Tin

WHAT TO DO:
1. Using a double glass boiler, heat the oil over hot water. If you prefer, you can heat oil in a pan directly over the burner on low heat or in a microwave until warm.
2. Add the beeswax and stir until melted.
3. Let oil cool slightly (not too long or it will set up).
4. Add the essential oils, starting with the base note, followed by the middle note, then the top note. Stir to blend.
5. Pour mixture into jars or tins immediately. If mixture begins to set, just reheat slightly.

TIP:
For variation, you can use solid coconut oil and omit the beeswax. You may also want to add 6-8 Vitamin E oil capsules as a preservative.

BASIC BATH OIL BLEND RECIPE

After a long day, soaking in a warm bath with a relaxing essential oil blend can be a delightful treat. Not only does it help take the edge off tense muscles, but it also ensures a better night's sleep. For early risers, starting your day with an invigorating essential oil blend at bath time may be more your speed, kick-starting your morning! Of course, a bath essential oil blend for achy joints can be helpful any time of day!

WHAT YOU WILL NEED:

1 cup Almond Oil or Coconut Oil

30 drops Top Note Essential Oil

20 drops Middle Note Essential Oil

10 drops Base Note Essential Oil

Corked container

Crystal beads, dried flowers, small seashells, etc. (Optional)

WHAT TO DO:

1. Pour the carrier oil through a funnel into the corked container, leaving about an inch at the top.

2. Add essential oils to container. Stir well to mix.

3. Cork the container and agitate the bottle gently.

4. Let it sit for 2-3 days before using. Add decor to your bottle.

5. For use, pour ½ - 1 teaspoon into the palm of your hand and gently massage into the body after a bath.

BASIC NASAL INHALER BLEND RECIPE

Filling a new nasal inhaler with your personal essential oil blend is an effective way to experience the therapeutic power of essential oils when suffering from emotional issues. Inhalers are also great to use for colds, flu, headaches, allergies, lung and chest congestion. They are small enough to carry in a pocket or purse and have on hand for immediate relief. Add 15-18 drops of your essential oil blend to your inhaler.

WHAT YOU WILL NEED:
9 drops Top Note Essential Oil
6 drops Middle Note Essential Oil
3 drops Base Note Essential Oil
Glass or Plastic Disposable Dropper
Small Plastic Inhaler

WHAT TO DO:
1. In a container, mix essential oils. Stir well to mix.
2. Use a glass or disposal dropper to fill nasal inhaler.
3. Carry and take a whiff as needed.

BASIC FOOT OIL BLEND RECIPE

A luxurious foot treatment with essential oils can readily deliver healing throughout the body. The sensitive skin and tissues of the feet take a lot of abuse and deserve a special blend that can easily be massaged in.

WHAT YOU WILL NEED:

1 ounce (30ml) Almond Oil

3 drops Top Note Essential Oil

2 drops Middle Note Essential Oil

1 drop Base Note Essential Oil

Plastic or Glass Bottle

WHAT TO DO:

1. In container, mix essential oils. Stir well to mix.
2. Add carrier oil to the bottle, replace lid and shake to blend.
3. To use, massage oil blend into feet after a bath or shower, or before bed. Wear soft, cotton socks to bed.

BASIC CAPSULE BLEND

Here is a simple recipe for making an essential oil capsule for ingestion. It is one of the best ways to take essential oils internally and bypass any unpleasant tastes. You can use 1-2 drops of essential oil per capsule (depending on size).

WHAT YOU WILL NEED:

1-2 drops Essential Oil* (20%)

Carrier Oil (80%)

WHAT TO DO:

1. Separate the two parts of the capsule. Remove the top half (wider cap). You will only be filling the bottom half.

2. Using a glass dropper, add essential oil one drop at a time directly into the capsule. This needs to be done carefully not to add too many drops or drip oil on the side of the capsule which will make it sticky.

3. Fill the remaining space with a carrier such as olive, coconut, pomegranate, etc.

4. Take the capsule immediately after filling it. These capsules will begin to dissolve right after filling.

5. Take one capsule once in the morning and once in the evening, or as prescribed by your healthcare provider.

*ONLY USE ESSENTIAL OILS THAT ARE SAFE TO INGEST.

BASIC BODY LOTION BLEND RECIPE

Do you want to try a good body lotion recipe? Why not make your own by following these simple instructions?

WHAT YOU WILL NEED:

4 ounces Unscented Lotion, Hydrosol and/or Carrier Oil
18 drops Top Note Essential Oil
12 drops Middle Note Essential Oil
6 drops Base Note Essential Oil
Plastic bottle or container

WHAT TO DO:

1. Add carrier oil to container.
2. Add essential oils starting with your base note essential oil first, followed by the middle note, and then the top note essential oil.
3. Recap and shake well to mix.
4. Use two to three times a day.

BASIC ROLL-ON OIL BLEND RECIPE

This basic recipe can be used to create a roll-on bottle applicator for your essential oil blend, depending on the oils you have on hand. Keep track of what you add or change, so you'll know how to make your favorite blends at a later time.

WHAT YOU WILL NEED:

½ ounce Jojoba Oil

9 drops Top Note Essential Oil

6 drops Middle Note Essential Oil

3 drops Base Note Essential Oil

Roll-on bottle

WHAT TO DO:

1. Add your carrier oil such as Jojoba to a roll-on bottle.
2. When adding essential oils, start with the base note and then add the middle note, followed by the top note. As you add each one, check the scent to make sure it is what you are looking for.
3. Insert the ball insert and apply 2-3 times a day.

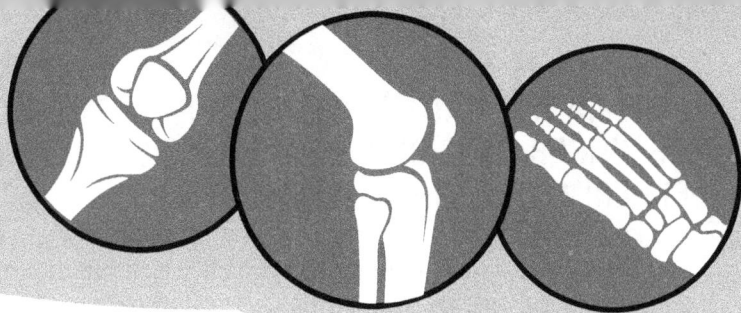

SUPPORTING RESEARCH

ANTI-INFLAMMATORY EFFECTS OF ESSENTIAL OILS OF GINGER (ZINGIBER OFFICINALE ROSECOE) IN EXPERIMENTAL RHEUMATOID ARTHRITIS

Author: Janet L. Funk, Jennifer B. Frye, Janice N. Oyarzo, Jianling Chen, Huaping Zhang, and Barbara N. Timmermann

Journal: Journal of PharmaNutrition. 2016 Jul;4(3):123-131

Location:

1. The University of Arizona, Tuscon, AZ, USA

2. The University of Kansas, Lawrence, KS, USA

Conclusion: Ginger's secondary metabolites (essential oils and gingerols) have anti-arthritic properties in the experimental model.

Abstract: Ginger and its extracts have been used traditionally as anti-inflammatory remedies, with a particular focus on the medicinal properties of its phenolic secondary metabolites, the gingerols. Consistent with these uses, potent anti-arthritic effects of gingerol-containing extracts were previously demonstrated by our laboratory using an experimental model of rheumatoid arthritis, streptococcal cell wall (SCW)-induced arthritis. In this study, anti-inflammatory effects of ginger's other secondary metabolites, the essential oils (GEO), which contain terpenes with reported phytoestrogenic activity, were assessed in female Lewis rats with SCW-induced arthritis. GEO (28 mg/kg/d ip) prevented chronic joint inflammation but altered neither the initial acute phase of joint swelling nor granuloma formation at sites of SCW deposition in the liver. Pharmacologic doses of 17-β estradiol (200 or 600 µg/kg/d sc) elicited the same pattern of anti-inflammatory activity, suggesting that GEO could be acting as a phytoestrogen. However, contrary to this hypothesis, GEO had no in vitro effect on classic estrogen target organs, such as uterus or bone. En toto, these results suggest that ginger's anti-inflammatory properties are not limited to the frequently studied phenolics, but may be attributable to the combined effects of both secondary metabolites, the pungent-tasting gingerols and as well as its aromatic essential oils.

ABERRANT HISTONE ACETYLATION CONTRIBUTES TO ELEVATED INTERLEUKIN-6 PRODUCTION IN RHEUMATOID ARTHRITIS SYNOVIAL FIBROBLASTS

Author: Wada TT, Araiki Y, Sato K, Aizaki Y, Yokota K, Kim YT, Oda H, Kurokawa R, and Mimura T

Journal: Journal of Biochem Biophys Res Commun. 2014 Feb 21;444(4):682-6

Location: Saitama Medical University, Saitama, Japan

Conclusion: IL-6 production is elevated in rheumatoid arthritis synovial fibroblasts.

Abstract: Accumulating evidence indicates that epigenetic aberrations have a role in the pathogenesis of rheumatoid arthritis (RA). However, reports on histone modifications are as yet quite limited in RA. Interleukin (IL)-6 is an inflammatory cytokine which is known to be involved in the pathogenesis of RA. Here we report the role of histone modifications in elevated IL-6 production in RA synovial fibroblasts (SFs). The level of histone H3 acetylation (H3ac) in the IL-6 promoter was significantly higher in RASFs than osteoarthritis (OA) SFs. This suggests that chromatin structure is in an open or loose state in the IL-6 promoter in RASFs. Furthermore, curcumin, a histone acetyltransferase (HAT) inhibitor, significantly reduced the level of H3ac in the IL-6 promoter, as well as IL-6 mRNA expression and IL-6 protein secretion by RASFs. Taken together, it is suggested that hyperacetylation of histone H3 in the IL-6 promoter induces the increase in IL-6 production by RASFs and thereby participates in the pathogenesis of RA.

ANTI-ARTHRITIC EFFECTS AND TOXICITY OF THE ESSENTIAL OILS OF TURMERIC (CURCUMA LONGA L.)

Author: Janet L. Funk, Jennifer B. Frye, Janice N. Oyarzo, Huaping Zhang, and Barbara N. Timmermann

Journal: Journal of J. Agric. Food Chem., 2010, 58 (2), pp 842–849

Location:

1. The University of Arizona, Tucson, Arizona

2. University of Kansas, Lawrence, Kansas

Conclusion: Researchers found that treatment with turmeric essential oil was 95 to 100 percent effective at preventing joint swelling in animals with induced arthritis.

Abstract: Turmeric (Curcuma longa L., Zingiberaceae) rhizomes contain two classes of secondary metabolites, curcuminoids, and the less well-studied essential oils. Having identified potent anti-arthritic effects of the curcuminoids in turmeric extracts in an animal model of rheumatoid arthritis (RA), studies were undertaken to determine whether the turmeric essential oils (TEO) were also joint protective using the same experimental model. Crude or refined TEO extracts dramatically inhibited joint swelling (90-100% inhibition) in female rats with streptococcal cell wall (SCW)-induced arthritis when extracts were administered via intraperitoneal injection to maximize uniform delivery. However, this anti-arthritic effect was accompanied by significant morbidity and mortality. Oral administration of a 20-fold higher dose TEO was non-toxic, but only mildly joint-protective (20% inhibition). These results do not support the isolated use of TEO for arthritis treatment, but, instead, identify potential safety concerns for invertebrates exposed to TEO.

BOSWELLIA FREREANA (FRANKINCENSE) SUPPRESSES CYTOKINE-INDUCED MATRIX METALLOPROTEINASE EXPRESSION AND PRODUCTION OF PRO-INFLAMMATORY MOLECULES IN ARTICULAR CARTILAGE

Author: Blain EJ, Ali AY, and Duance VC

Journal: Journal of Phytother Res. 2010 Jun;24(6):905-12

Location: Cardiff University, Cardiff, United Kingdom

Conclusion: The efficacy of Boswellia frereana extracts potential benefits for treating osteoarthritis.

Abstract: This study aimed to assess the anti-inflammatory efficacy of Boswellia frereana extracts in an in vitro model of cartilage degeneration and determine its potential as a therapy for treating osteoarthritis. Cartilage degradation was induced in vitro by treating explants with 5 ng/ml interleukin1alpha (IL-1alpha) and 10 ng/ml oncostatin M (OSM) over a 28-day period, in the presence or absence of 100 micro g/ml B. frereana. Treatment of IL-1alpha/OSM stimulated cartilage explants with B. frereana inhibited the breakdown of the collagenous matrix. B. frereana reduced MMP9 and MMP13 mRNA levels, inhibited MMP9 expression and activation, and significantly reduced the production of nitrite (the stable end product of nitric oxide), prostaglandin E2 and cyclooxygenase-2. Epi-lupeol was identified as the principal constituent of B. frereana. This is the first report on the novel anti-inflammatory properties of Boswellia frereana in an in vitro model of cartilage degradation. We have demonstrated that B. frereana prevents collagen degradation, and inhibits the production of pro-inflammatory mediators and MMPs. Due to its efficacy, we propose that B. frereana should be examined further as a potential therapeutic agent for treating inflammatory symptoms associated with arthritis.

FRANKINCENSE AND MYRRH SUPPRESS INFLAMMATION VIA REGULATION OF THE METABOLIC PROFILING AND THE MAPK SIGNALING PATHWAY

Author: Shulan Su, Jinao Duan, Ting Chen, Xiaochen Huang, Erxin Shang, Li Yu, Keifeng Wei, Yue Zhu, Jianming Guo, Sheng Guo, Pei Liu, Dawei Qian, and Yuping Tang

Journal: Journal of Sci Rep. 2015; 5: 13668

Location: Nanjing University of Chinese Medicine, Nanjing, China

Conclusion: Frankincense and myrrh are highly effective in the treatment of inflammatory diseases.

Abstract: Frankincense and myrrh are highly effective in the treatment of inflammatory diseases, but lacking the therapy mechanisms. We undertook this study to evaluate the effects on Adjuvant-induced Arthritis (AIA) rats and to explore the underlying mechanisms by analyzing the metabolic profiling and signaling pathway evaluated by expression of inflammatory cytokines, c-jun and c-fos and corresponding phosphorylation levels. The results stated the elevated expression levels of TNFα, PGE2, IL-2, NO, and MDA in serum and swelling paw of AIA rats were significantly decreased after treatment, which exerted more remarkable inhibitive effects of combined therapy. The metabolic profiling of plasma and urine were clearly improved, and twenty-one potential biomarkers were identified. Moreover, the inhibited effects of five bioactive components on cytokine transcription in PHA stimulated-PBMC showed the MAPK pathway might account for this phenomenon with a considerable reduction in phosphorylated forms of all the three MAPK (ERK1/2, p38, and JNK) and down-regulation of c-jun and c-fos.

CHEMICAL COMPOSITION, ANTIOXIDANT, ANTI-INFLAMMATORY AND ANTI-PROLIFERATIVE ACTIVITIES OF ESSENTIAL OILS OF PLANTS FROM BURKINA FASO

Author: Bagora Bayala, Imaël Henri Nestor Bassole, Charlemagne Gnoula, Roger Nebie, Albert Yonli, Laurent Morel, Gilles Figueredo, Jean-Baptiste Nikiema, Jean-Marc A. Lobaccaro, and Jacques Simpore

Journal: Journal of PLoS One. 2014; 9(3): e92122

Location:

1. Université de Ouagadougou, Ouagadougou, Burkina Faso

2. Clermont Université, Université Blaise Pascal, Génétique Reproduction et Développement (GReD), Clermont-Ferrand, France

3. Centre National de la Recherche Scientifique (CNRS), Unité Mixte de Recherche (UMR) 6293, GReD, Aubière, France

4. Institut National de la Santé et de la Recherche Médicale (INSERM), UMR 1103, GReD, Aubière, France

5. Centre de Recherche en Nutrition Humaine d'Auvergne, Clermont-Ferrand, France

6. LEXVA Analytique, Biopole Clermont-Limagne, Saint-Beauzire, France

7. Institut de Génomique Fonctionnelle de Lyon, France

Conclusion: Shows ginger and basil essential oils have anti-inflammatory properties used to help relieve arthritis pain.

Abstract: This research highlights the chemical composition, antioxidant, anti-inflammatory and antiproliferative activities of essential oils from leaves of Ocimum basilicum, Ocimum americanum, Hyptis spicigera, Lippia multiflora, Ageratum conyzoides, Eucalyptus camaldulensis, and Zingiber officinale. Essential oils were analyzed by gas chromatography-mass spectrometry and gas chromatography-flame ionization detector. Major constituents were α-terpineol (59.78%) and β-caryophyllene (10.54%) for Ocimum basilicum; 1, 8-cineol (31.22%), camphor (12.730%), α-pinene (6.87%) and trans α-bergamotene (5.32%) for Ocimum americanum; β-caryophyllene (21%), α-pinene (20.11%), sabinene (10.26%), β-pinene (9.22%) and α-phellandrene (7.03%) for Hyptis spicigera; p-cymene

(25.27%), β-caryophyllene (12.70%), thymol (11.88), γ-terpinene (9.17%) and thymyle acetate (7.64%) for Lippia multiflora; precocene (82.10%) for Ageratum conyzoides; eucalyptol (59.55%), α-pinene (9.17%) and limonene (8.76%) for Eucalyptus camaldulensis; arcurcumene (16.67%), camphene (12.70%), zingiberene (8.40%), β-bisabolene (7.83%) and β-sesquiphellandrène (5.34%) for Zingiber officinale. Antioxidant activities were examined using 1,1-diphenyl-2-picryl-hydrazyl (DPPH) and 2,2′-azinobis-(3-ethylbenzothiazoline-6-sulfonic acid (ABTS) methods. O. basilicum and L. multiflora exhibited the highest antioxidant activity in DPPH and ABTS tests, respectively. Anti-inflammatory properties were evaluated by measuring the inhibition of lipoxygenase activity, and essential oil of Z. officinale was the most active. The anti-proliferative effect was assayed by the measurement of MTT on LNCaP and PC-3 prostate cancer cell lines, and SF-763 and SF-767 glioblastoma cell lines. Essential oils from A. conyzoides and L. multiflora were the most active on LNCaP and PC-3 cell lines, respectively. The SF-767 glioblastoma cell line was the most sensitive to O. basilicum and L. multiflora EOs while essential oil of A. conyzoides showed the highest activity on SF-763 cells. Altogether these results justify the use of these plants in traditional medicine in Burkina Faso and open a new field of investigation in the characterization of the molecules involved in anti-proliferative processes.

EFFECT OF EUCALYPTUS OIL INHALATION ON PAIN AND INFLAMMATORY RESPONSES AFTER TOTAL KNEE REPLACEMENT: A RANDOMIZED CLINICAL TRIAL.

Author: Jun YS, Kang P, Min SS, Lee JM, Kim HK, Seol GH

Journal: Journal of Evidence-Based Complementary and Alternative Medicine Volume 2013, Article ID 502727, 7 pages

Location: Korea University, Seoul, Republic of Korea

Conclusion: Eucalyptus oil has been reported effective in reducing pain, swelling, and inflammation after total knee replacement surgery.

Abstract: Eucalyptus oil has been reported effective in reducing pain, swelling, and inflammation. This study aimed to investigate the effects of eucalyptus oil inhalation on pain and inflammatory responses after total knee replacement (TKR) surgery. Participants were randomized 1:1 to the intervention group (eucalyptus inhalation group) or control group (almond oil inhalation group). Patients inhaled eucalyptus or almond oil for 30 min of continuous passive motion (CPM) on 3 consecutive days. Pain on a visual analog scale (VAS), blood pressure, heart rate, C-reactive protein (CRP) concentration, and white blood cell (WBC) count were measured before and after inhalation. Pain VAS on all three days ($P <$ .001) and systolic ($P < .05$) and diastolic ($P = .03$) blood pressure on the second day were significantly lower in the group inhaling eucalyptus than that inhaling almond oil. Heart rate, CRP, and WBC, however, did not differ significantly in the two groups. In conclusion, inhalation of eucalyptus oil was effective in decreasing patient's pain and blood pressure following TKR, suggesting that eucalyptus oil inhalation may be a nursing intervention for the relief of pain after TKR.

EFFICACY OF TURMERIC EXTRACTS AND CURCUMIN FOR ALLEVIATING THE SYMPTOMS OF JOINT ARTHRITIS: A SYSTEMATIC REVIEW AND META-ANALYSIS OF RANDOMIZED CLINICAL TRIALS.

Author: Daily JW, Yang M, and Park S

Journal: Journal of J Med Food. 2016 Aug;19(8):717-29

Location:

1. Department of R&D Daily Manufacturing, Inc., Rockwell, North Carolina, USA

2. Hoseo University, Asan, South Korea

Conclusion: Turmeric extract appears to reduce symptoms of arthritis.

Abstract: Although turmeric and its curcumin-enriched extracts have been used for treating arthritis, no systematic review and meta-analysis of randomized clinical trials (RCTs) have been conducted to evaluate the strength of the research. We systemically evaluated all RCTs of turmeric extracts and curcumin for treating arthritis symptoms to elucidate the efficacy of curcuma for alleviating the symptoms of arthritis. Literature searches were conducted using 12 electronic databases, including PubMed, Embase, Cochrane Library, Korean databases, Chinese medical databases, and Indian scientific database. Search terms used were "turmeric," "curcuma," "curcumin," "arthritis," and "osteoarthritis." A pain visual analogue score (PVAS) and Western Ontario and McMaster Universities Osteoarthritis Index (WOMAC) were used for the significant outcomes of arthritis. Initial searches yielded 29 articles, of which 8 met specific selection criteria. Three among the included RCTs reported reduction of PVAS (mean difference: −2.04 [−2.85, −1.24]) with turmeric/curcumin in comparison with placebo (P < .00001), whereas meta-analysis of four studies showed a decrease of WOMAC with turmeric/curcumin treatment (mean difference: −15.36 [−26.9, −3.77]; P = .009). Furthermore, there was no significant mean difference in PVAS between turmeric/curcumin and pain medicine in a meta-analysis of five studies. Eight RCTs included in the review exhibited low to moderate risk of bias. There was no publication bias in the meta-analysis. In conclusion, these RCTs provide scientific evidence that supports the efficacy of turmeric extract (about 1000 mg/ day of curcumin) in the treatment of arthritis. However, the total number of RCTs included in the analysis, the total sample size, and the methodological quality of the primary studies were not sufficient to draw definitive conclusions. Thus, more rigorous and more extensive studies are needed to confirm the therapeutic efficacy of turmeric for arthritis.

ANTI-ARTHRITIC EFFECTS AND TOXICITY OF THE ESSENTIAL OILS OF TURMERIC (CURCUMA LONGA L.)

Author: Funk JL, Frye JB, Oyarzo JN, Zhang H, Timmermann BN

Journal: Journal of J Agric Food Chem. 2010 Jan 27;58(2):842-9

Location: University of Arizona, Tucson, Arizona, USA

Conclusion: Turmeric essential oils reduced joint inflammation in rats.

Abstract: Turmeric (Curcuma longa L., Zingiberaceae) rhizomes contain two classes of secondary metabolites, curcuminoids, and the less well-studied essential oils. Having previously identified potent anti-arthritic effects of the curcuminoids in turmeric extracts in an animal model of rheumatoid arthritis (RA), studies were undertaken to determine whether the turmeric essential oils (TEO) were also joint protective using the same experimental model. Crude or refined TEO extracts dramatically inhibited joint swelling (90-100% inhibition) in female rats with streptococcal cell wall (SCW)-induced arthritis when extracts were administered via intraperitoneal injection to maximize uniform delivery. However, this anti-arthritic effect was accompanied by significant morbidity and mortality. Oral administration of a 20-fold higher dose TEO was nontoxic, but only mildly joint-protective (20% inhibition). These results do not support the isolated use of TEO for arthritis treatment but, instead, identify potential safety concerns for invertebrates exposed to TEO.

BIOLOGICAL ACTIVITIES AND SAFETY OF CITRUS SPP. ESSENTIAL OILS

Author: Noura S. Dosoky and William N. Setzer

Journal: Journal of Int J Mol Sci. 2018 Jul; 19(7): 1966

Location: University of Alabama, Huntsville, USA

Conclusion: This review summarizes the important biological activities and safety concerns of orange.

Abstract: Citrus fruits have been a commercially important crop for thousands of years. Also, Citrus essential oils are valuable in the perfume, food, and beverage industries, and have also enjoyed use as aromatherapy and medicinal agents. This review summarizes the important biological activities and safety considerations of the essential oils of sweet orange (Citrus sinensis), bitter orange (Citrus aurantium), neroli (Citrus aurantium), orange petitgrain (Citrus aurantium), mandarin (Citrus reticulata), lemon (Citrus limon), lime (Citrus aurantifolia), grapefruit (Citrus × paradisi), bergamot (Citrus bergamia), Yuzu (Citrus junos), and kumquat (Citrus japonica).

THYMUS MASTICHINA L. ESSENTIAL OILS FROM MURCIA (SPAIN): COMPOSITION AND ANTIOXIDANT, ANTIENZYMATIC AND ANTIMICROBIAL BIOACTIVITIES

Author: Ana-Belen Cutillas, Alejandro Carrasco, Ramiro Martinez-Gutierrez, Virginia Tomas, Jose Tudela, and Gebriel Agbor

Journal: Journal of PLoS One. 2018; 13(1): e0190790

Location:

1. University of Murica, Murica, Spain

2. Novozymes Spain S.A., Madrid, Spain

Conclusion: Bornyl acetate and limonene showed the highest lipoxygenase inhibition, and 1,8-cineole was the best acetylcholinesterase inhibitor. Moreover, these EOs inhibited the growth of Escherichia coli, Staphylococcus aureus and Candida albicans due to the contribution of their individual compounds.

Abstract: The compositions of essential oils (EOs) from Spanish marjoram (Thymus mastichina L.) grown in several bioclimatic zones of Murcia (SE Spain) were studied to determine their absolute and relative concentrations using gas chromatography-mass spectrometry. 1,8-Cineole and linalool were the main components, followed by α-pinene, β-pinene, and α-terpineol. (−)-Linalool, (+)-α-terpineol and (+)-α-pinene were the most abundant enantiomers. When the antioxidant capacities of T. mastichina EOs and their compounds were measured by five methods, EOs and linalool, linalyl acetate, α-terpinene, and γ-terpinene, among others, showed antioxidant activities. All four T. mastichina EOs inhibited both lipoxygenase and acetylcholinesterase activities, and they might be useful for further research into inflammatory and Alzheimer diseases. Bornyl acetate and limonene showed the highest lipoxygenase inhibition and 1,8-cineole was the best acetylcholinesterase inhibitor. Moreover, these EOs inhibited the growth of Escherichia coli, Staphylococcus aureus and Candida albicans due to the contribution of their individual compounds. The results underline the potential use of these EOs in manufactured products, such as foodstuff, cosmetics, and pharmaceuticals.

THE EFFECTIVENESS OF AROMATHERAPY IN REDUCING PAIN: A SYSTEMATIC REVIEW AND META-ANALYSIS

Author: Shaheen E. Lakhan, Heather Sheafer, and Deborah Tepper

Journal: Journal of Pain Res Treat. 2016; 2016: 8158693

Location:

1. Global Neuroscience Initiative Foundation, Los Angeles, CA, USA

2. California University of Science and Medicine, Colton, CA, USA

3. Neurological Institute, Cleveland Clinic, Cleveland, OH, USA

Conclusion: There is a significant positive effect of aromatherapy (compared to placebo or treatments as usual controls) in reducing pain reported on a visual analog scale.

Abstract: Aromatherapy refers to the medicinal or therapeutic use of essential oils absorbed through the skin or olfactory system. Recent literature has examined the effectiveness of aromatherapy in treating pain.

Method: 12 studies examining the use of aromatherapy for pain management were identified through an electronic database search. A meta-analysis was performed to determine the effects of aromatherapy on pain.

Results: There is a significant positive effect of aromatherapy (compared to placebo or treatments as usual controls) in reducing pain reported on a visual analog scale (SMD = -1.18, 95% CI: -1.33, -1.03; $p < 0.0001$). Secondary analyses found that aromatherapy is more consistent for treating nociceptive (SMD = -1.57, 95% CI: -1.76, -1.39, $p < 0.0001$) and acute pain (SMD = -1.58, 95% CI: -1.75, -1.40, $p < 0.0001$) than inflammatory (SMD = -0.53, 95% CI: -0.77, -0.29, $p < 0.0001$) and chronic pain (SMD = -0.22, 95% CI: -0.49, 0.05, $p = 0.001$), respectively. Based on the available research, aromatherapy is most effective in treating postoperative pain (SMD = -1.79, 95% CI: -2.08, -1.51, $p < 0.0001$) and obstetrical and gynecological pain (SMD = -1.14, 95% CI: -2.10, -0.19, $p < 0.0001$).

Conclusion: The findings of this study indicate that aromatherapy can successfully treat pain when combined with conventional treatments.

COMPARISON OF THE EFFECT OF TOPICAL APPLICATION OF ROSEMARY AND MENTHOL FOR MUSCULOSKELETAL PAIN IN HEMODIALYSIS PATIENTS

Author: Sekine Keshavarzian and Nahid Shahgholian

Journal: Journal of Iran J Nurs Midwifery Res. 2017 Nov-Dec; 22(6): 436–441

Location: Isfahan University of Medical Sciences, Isfahan, Iran

Conclusion: Topical application of menthol and rosemary can alleviate the severity and frequency of recurrence of musculoskeletal pain in hemodialysis patients; however, according to the results of the study, none had precedence over the other.

Abstract: Pain is the most common problem experienced by hemodialysis patients, especially musculoskeletal pain in lower extremities, which is usually not wholly treated and adversely affects their quality of life. The present study was conducted with the aim to determine and compare the effects of topical application of menthol and rosemary for musculoskeletal pain in hemodialysis patients.

Materials and Methods: The present single-blind clinical trial recruited 105 eligible patients undergoing hemodialysis in selected hospitals affiliated to Isfahan University of Medical Sciences; patients were selected by convenient sampling. Participants' severity of pain was determined prior to intervention. They were then randomly divided into rosemary, menthol, and placebo groups. All three groups applied medication on the site of pain on their legs three times a day for three days and recorded the severity of pain four hours after morning and afternoon applications. The statistical analysis of data was performed using SPSS 18.

Results: The mean score of severity of pain before the intervention was not significantly different among the three groups (p = 0.83), but it became significantly different after intervention (p = 0.001). Significant differences were observed in mean severity of pain before and after intervention in rosemary and menthol groups (p < 0.001), but not in the placebo group (p = 0.21).

Conclusion: Topical application of menthol and rosemary can alleviate the severity and frequency of recurrence of musculoskeletal pain in hemodialysis patients; however, according to the results of the study, none had precedence over the other.

EFFECT OF LAVENDER (LAVANDULA ANGUSTIFOLIA) ESSENTIAL OIL ON ACUTE INFLAMMATORY RESPONSE

Author: Gabriel Fernando Esteves Cardia, Saulo Euclides Silva-Filho, Expedito Leite Silva, Nancy Sayuri Uchida, Heitor Augusto Otaviano Cavalcante, Larissa Laila Cassarotti, Valter Eduardo Cocco Salvadego, Ricardo Alexandre Spironello, Ciomar Aparecida Bersani-Amado, and Roberto Kenji Nakamura Cuman

Journal: Journal of Evid Based Complement Alternat Med. 2018; 2018: 1413940

Location:

1. Federal University of Grande Dourados, Dourados, MS, Brazil

2. State University of Maringá, Maringá, PR, Brazil

Conclusion: In this study, Lavandula angustifolia was evaluated for its positive effect on acute inflammation.

Abstract: Lavandula angustifolia is a plant of Lamiaceae family, with many therapeutic properties and biological activities, such as anticonvulsant, anxiolytic, antioxidant, anti-inflammatory, and antimicrobial activities. This study aimed to evaluate the effect of Lavandula angustifolia Mill. Essential oil (LEO) on the acute inflammatory response. LEO was analyzed using gas chromatography-mass spectrometry (GC-MS) and nuclear magnetic resonance spectroscopy (NMR) methods and showed a predominance of 1,8-cineole (39.83%), borneol (22.63%), and camphor (22.12%). LEO at concentrations of 0.5, 1, 3, and 10 µg/ml did not present in vitro cytotoxicity. Additionally, LEO did not stimulate the leukocyte chemotaxis in vitro. The LEO topical application at concentrations of 0.25, 0.5, and 1 mg/ear reduced edema formation, myeloperoxidase (MPO) activity, and nitric oxide (NO) production in croton oil-induced ear edema model. In carrageenan-induced paw edema model, LEO treatment at doses of 75, 100, and 250 mg/kg reduced edema formation, MPO activity, and NO production. In dextran-induced paw edema model, LEO at doses of 75 and 100 mg/kg reduced paw edema and MPO activity. In conclusion, LEO presented anti-inflammatory activity, and the mechanism proposed of LEO seems to be, at least in part, involving the participation of prostanoids, NO, proinflammatory cytokines, and histamine.

ZINGIBER OFFICINALE: A POTENTIAL PLANT AGAINST RHEUMATOID ARTHRITIS

Author: Abdullah Al-Nahain, Rownak Jahan, and Mohammed Rahmatullah

Journal: Journal of Arthritis. 2014; 2014: 159089

Location: University of Development Alternative, Dhaka, Bangladesh

Conclusion: Symptomatic relief from ginger essential oil from RA-induced bone destruction.

Abstract: Rheumatoid arthritis (RA) is an autoimmune disease particularly affecting elderly people which leads to massive bone destruction with consequent inflammation, pain, and disability. Allopathic medicine can provide only symptomatic relief. However, Zingiber officinale is a plant belonging to the Zingiberaceae family, which has traditionally been used for the treatment of RA in alternative medicines of many countries. Many of the phytochemical constituents of the rhizomes of this plant have therapeutic benefits including amelioration of RA. This review attempts to list those phytochemical constituents with their reported mechanisms of action. It is concluded that these phytochemicals can form the basis of the discovery of new drugs, which not only can provide symptomatic relief but also may provide total relief from RA by stopping RA-induced bone destruction. As the development of RA is a complex process, further research should be continued towards elucidating the molecular details leading to RA and drugs that can stop or reverse these processes by phytoconstituents of ginger.

THE EFFECTS OF AROMATHERAPY ON PAIN, DEPRESSION, AND LIFE SATISFACTION OF ARTHRITIS PATIENTS

Author: Kim MJ, Nam ES, and Paik SL

Journal: Journal of Taehan Kanho Hakhoe Chi. 2005 Feb;35(1):186-94

Location: The Catholic University of Korea, Korea

Conclusion: The result of this study clearly shows that aromatherapy has major effects on decreasing pain and depression levels. Based on our experiment's findings, we suggest that aromatherapy can be a useful nursing intervention for arthritis patients.

Purpose: The purpose of this study was to investigate the effect of aromatherapy on pain, depression, and feelings of satisfaction in the life of arthritis patients.

Method: This study used a quasi-experimental design with a non-equivalent control group, pre-and post-test. The sample consisted of 40 patients, enrolled in the Rheumatics Center, Kangnam St. Mary's Hospital, South Korea. The essential oils used were lavender, marjoram, eucalyptus, rosemary, and peppermint blended in proportions of 2:1:2:1:1. They were mixed with a carrier oil composed of almond (45%), apricot(45%), and jojoba oil(10%) and they were diluted to 1.5% after blending. The data were analyzed using a 2-test, Fisher's exact test, t-test, and paired t-test.

Result: Aromatherapy significantly decreased both the pain score and the depression score of the experimental group compared with the control group. However, aromatherapy didn't increase the feeling of satisfaction in the life of the experimental group compared with the control group.

HEALING ARTHRITIS NATURALLY WITH ESSENTIAL OIL

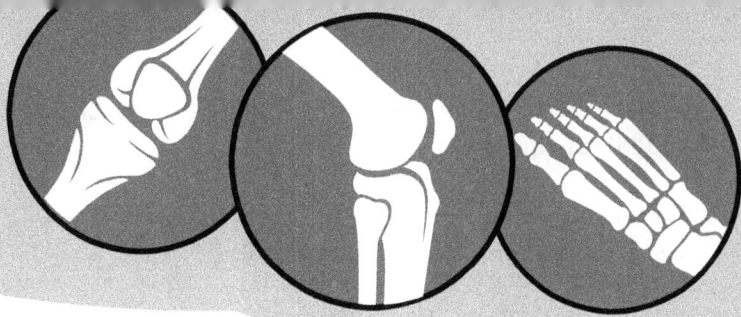

BIBLIOGRAPHY

The Encyclopedia of Essential Oils: The Complete Guide to the Use of Aromatic Oils in Aromatherapy, Herbalism, Health & Well Being, by Julia Lawless

Medical Aromatherapy: Healing with Essential Oils, by Kurt Schnaubelt, Ph.D.

The Art of Aromatherapy: The Healing and Beautifying Properties of the Essential Oils of Flowers and Herbs, by Robert B. Tisserand

The Encyclopedia of Aromatherapy, by Chrissie Wildwood

The Complete Book of Essential Oils and Aromatherapy, by Valerie Ann Worwood

The Aromatherapy Encyclopedia: A Concise Guide to Over 385 Plant Oils, by Carol Schiller and David Schiller

Aromatherapy: An A-Z: The Most Comprehensive Guide to Aromatherapy Ever Published, by Patricia Davis

Clinical Aromatherapy: Essential Oils In Practice, 2nd edition, by Jane Buckle

Aromatherapy: A Complete Guide to the Healing Art, 2nd edition, by Kathi Keville and Mindy Green

Hands-On Healing Remedies: 150 Recipes for Herbal Balms, Salves, Oils, Liniments, and other Topical Therapies, by Stephanie L. Tourles

375 Essential Oils and Hydrosols, by Jeanne Rose

Organic Beauty with Essential Oil: For Natural Skin Care, Hair Care and Bath & Body Products, by Rebecca Park Totilo

Therapeutic Blending With Essential Oil: Decoding the Healing Matrix of Aromatherapy, by Rebecca Park Totilo

The Healing Intelligence of Essential Oils: The Science of Advanced Aromatherapy, by Kurt Schnaubelt, Ph.D.

The Encyclopedia of Aromatherapy, by Chrissie Wildwood

Muhlbauer RC, Lozano A., Palacio S. et al. Common herbs, essential oils, and monoterpenes potently modulate bone metabolism. *Bone*. 2003 Apr.32(4);372-80

Metin, ZG, OZdemir, L. The Effects of Aromatherapy Massage and Reflexology on Pain and Fatigue in Patients with Rheumatoid Arthritis: A Randomized Controlled Trial. Pain Management Nursing official journal of the American Society of Pain Management Nurses 17(2). April 2016;991

Essential Oil Safety 2nd Edition by Robert Tisserand and Rodney Young

Modern Essentials 10th Edition, by Aroma Tools

Essential Oils Desk Reference 7th Edition, by Life Science Publishing

Evidence-Based Essential Oil Therapy: The Ultimate Guide to the Therapeutic and Clinical Application of Essential Oils by Dr. Scott A. Johnson

The Chemistry of Aromatherapeutic Oils by E. Joy Bowles

Essential Chemistry for Aromatherapy by Sue Clarke

National Center for Biotechnology Information, US National Library of Medicine and National Institutes of Health

OTHER BOOKS
BY
REBECCA PARK TOTILO

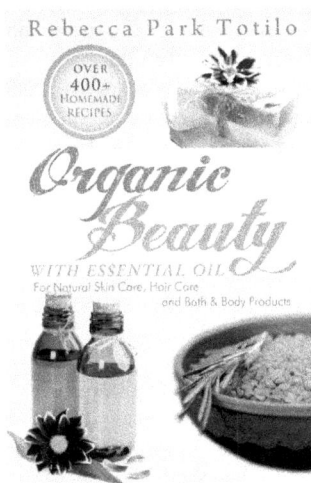

Organic Beauty With Essential Oil: Over 400+ Homemade Recipes for Natural Skin Care, Hair Care and Bath & Body Products

Sweep aside all those harmful chemically-based cosmetics and make your own organic bath and body products at home with the magic of potent essential oils! In this book, you'll find a luxurious array of over 400 Eco-friendly recipes that call for breathtaking fragrances and soothing, rich organic ingredients satisfying you head to toe. Included you'll find helpful can have the confidence knowing which essential oil to use and how much when creating your own body scrub, lip butter, or lotion bar! Discover how easy it is to make bath treats like fragrant shower gels, dreamy bubble baths, luscious creams and lotions, deep cleansing masks and facials for literally pennies using only a few essential oils and ingredients from your own kitchen with Organic Beauty with Essential Oil.

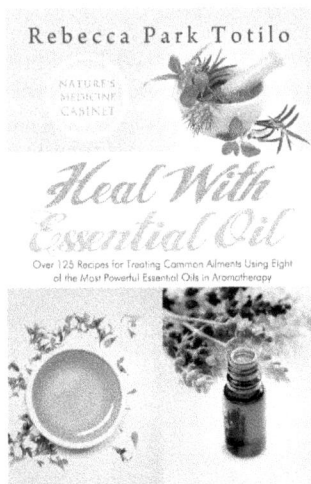

Heal With Essential Oil: Nature's Medicine Cabinet

Using essential oils drawn from nature's own medicine cabinet of flowers, trees, seeds and roots, man can tap into God's healing power to heal oneself from almost any pain. Find relief from many conditions and rejuvenate the body. With over 125 recipes, this practical guide will walk you through in the most easy-to-understand form how to treat common ailments with your essential oils for everyday living. Filled with practical advice on therapeutic blending of oils and safety, a directory of the most effective oils for common ailments and easy to follow remedies chart, and prescriptive blends for aches, pains and sicknesses.

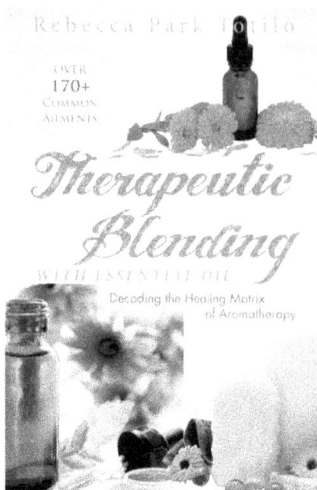

Therapeutic Blending With Essential Oil: Decoding the Healing Matrix of Aromatherapy

Therapeutic Blending With Essential Oil unlocks the healing power of essential oils and guides you through the intricate matrix of aromatherapy, with a compilation of over 170 common ailments. Discover how to properly formulate a blend for any physical or emotional symptom with easy to follow customizable recipes. Now, you can make your own personalized massage oils, hand and body lotions, bath gels, compresses, salve ointments, smelling salts, nasal inhalers and more. This exhaustive guide takes all the guesswork out of blending essential oils from how many drops to include in a blend, to working with and measuring thick oils, to how often to apply it for acute or chronic conditions. It also shows you how to create a single blend for multiple conditions. Even if you run out of oil for a favorite recipe, this book shows you how to substitute it with another oil.

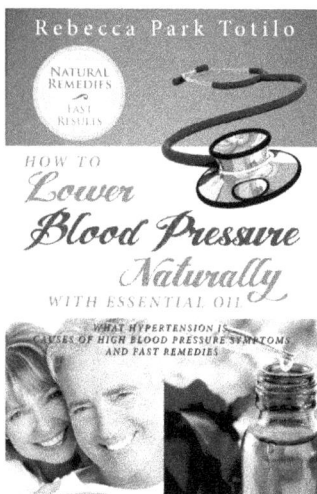

How To Lower Blood Pressure Naturally With Essential Oil: What Hypertension Is, Causes of High Pressure Symptoms and Fast Remedies

One out of three adults have it, and another one-third don't realize it. Oftentimes, it goes undetected for years. Even those who take multiple medications for it still don't have it under control. It's no secret -- high blood pressure is rampant in America. High blood pressure, or hypertension, has become a household term. Between balancing meds and monitoring diets though, are the true causes -- and best treatments -- hidden in the shadows? In How to Lower Blood Pressure Naturally With Essential Oil, Rebecca Park Totilo sheds light on what high blood pressure is, the causes and symptoms of high blood pressure, and which essential oils regulate blood pressure and how to use essential oils as a natural, alternative method.

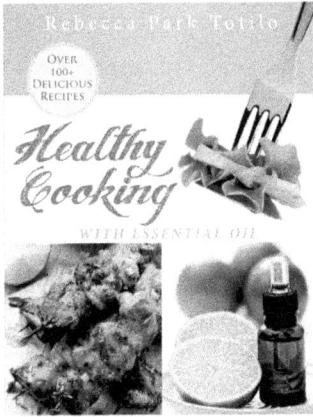

Healthy Cooking with Essential Oil

Imagine transforming an everyday dish into something extraordinary using only a drop or two of essential oil can enliven everything from soups, salads, to main dishes and desserts. Boasting flavor and fragrance, these intense essences can turn a dull, boring meal into something appetizing and delicious. Essential oils are fun, easy-to-use and beneficial, compared to the traditional stale, dried herbs and spices found in most pantries today. Healthy food should never be thought of as mere fuel for the body, it should be enjoyed as a multi-sensory experience that brings therapeutic value as well as nourishment. For years we have limited the use of essential oils to scented candles and soaps, in the belief that they were unsafe to consume (and some are!). However, more people are realizing the value of using pure essential oils to enhance their diet. In Healthy Cooking With Essential Oil, you will learn how cooking with essential oils can open up a wealth of creative opportunities in the kitchen.

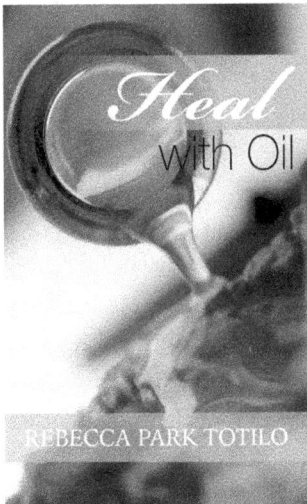

Heal With Oil: How to Use the Essential Oils of Ancient Scripture

During ancient times, spices, resins and other aromatics were an integral part of the Hebraic culture. People of the Holy Land understood the use of fragrant plants in maintaining wellness and physical healing, as well as the plant's oil to enhance their spiritual state in worship, prayer and confession, and for cleansing and purification from sin. Since the creation, fragrant oils have been inhaled, applied to the body, and taken internally in which the benefits extended to every aspect of their being. Buried within the passages of scriptures lies a hidden treasure – possibly every man's answer to illness and disease. Now you can learn their secret and discover how to transform your life and walk in divine health.

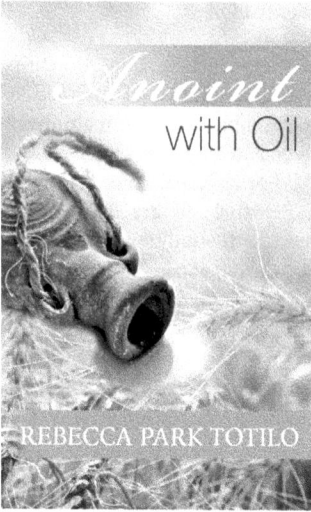

Anoint with Oil

If you were taught by church leaders that anointing with oil ceased during Old Testament times, or that it is simply "symbolic" and has no power or significance today, you may be missing beauty and depth in your spiritual journey. Anointing with oil brings real benefits into your life, such as promotion, discernment, sensitivity, fruitfulness, and declaration. In Anoint With Oil, Rebecca Park Totilo shares an aromatic and sacred expedition through the scriptures, showing the purpose of anointing with oil, the methods used in the Bible and their symbolism, the ingredients of the holy anointing oil, and the uses of essential oils mentioned in the Old and New Testaments. Discover new scents within these pages and find out: – Why the right ear, right thumb, and right big toe? – What is the mysterious fifth ingredient of the holy anointing oil? – Which oils did Jesus anoint with? – Who performs the anointing ritual? – How can I benefit from anointing with oil?

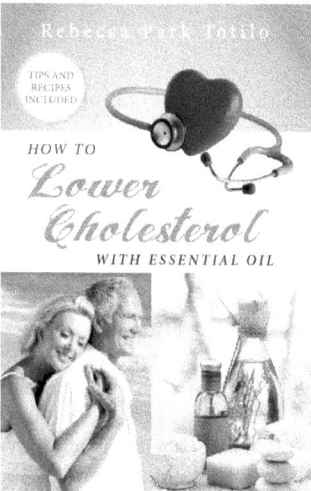

How to Lower Cholesterol with Essential Oil

Take healthy steps now to control high cholesterol and its risk factors with essential oils. People with high cholesterol have twice the risk for heart disease according to the Center for Disease Control and Prevention. What's worse, most folks aren't even aware that they have atherosclerosis until they have a heart attack or stroke. Lowering your cholesterol and triglycerides with essential oils may slow, reduce, or even stop the buildup of dangerous plaque in your arteries causing blockage of blood flow which could result in a heart attack or stroke. In this indispensable guide, author Rebecca Park Totilo presents scientific research supporting the efficacy of certain essential oils for lowering cholesterol, an extensive essential oil and carrier oil directory, natural treatments with recipes, along with easy-to-follow methods of use via inhalation, topically, and ingestion.

www.ingramcontent.com/pod-product-compliance
Lightning Source LLC
Chambersburg PA
CBHW071131280326
41935CB00010B/1185